A

MW01274888

From Birth to Puberty

"I thoroughly recommend this book to anyone who has children. The earlier parents read it the better. It is a great way to be prepared for all those moments which happen in life with children. If you want your child to be successful in their relationships as they grow up read *From Birth to Puberty*. Children learn from watching their parents, and this book will be a great help as you apply it to your own understanding and therefore the understanding of your children."

-Sue Bagshaw , Senior Doctor, Christchurch Youth Health Centre
President, International Association for Adolescent Health
Senior Lecturer, University of Otago

"A useful, friendly, inclusive and positive book covering an important area of education. I love the inclusive language used. I would recommend the book without hesitation. It covers the entire range of experience termed 'sexuality' in a way that is empowering, comprehensive and holistic. We would put it on our bookshelves at Playcentres very happily."

-Tess Conran-Liew, Psychologist, New Zealand Playcentre Federation

"...a book which will be invaluable to parents and caregivers in guiding their children to becoming healthy adults, comfortable with their sexuality. Having worked extensively with adolescents, I believe that many of their problems would not have occured if they had a 'matter of fact' open and honest relationship with their parents such as this book models. I recommend this book to parents as a very necessary resource."

- Joan Plowman BN, Coordinator, Child Health Programme,
Hawke's Bay District Health Board

"I see this book as enabling parents to handle the complex tasks of parenting with more confidence. The case histories throughout *From Birth to Puberty* help parents relate to situations in a sympathetic way. Above all it is a very practical book with lots of creative ideas to stimulate parents rather than make them feel guilty about things they have or haven't done."

-Margaret Sparrow MBE, Sexual Health Physician

"Parents will find this book informative and easy to read. It covers a broad range of issues, and our Preschool Management Advisers think that including experiences and examples is a great idea - first hand knowledge for parents - ie easy to relate to. For a topic that is sometimes awkward or embarrassing for parents it covers issues in a relaxing and easy going manner."

-Kindergarten Parents Victoria

"In my job I get the chance to read and recommend many books on sex and sexuality and I do not hesitate to recommend *From Birth to Puberty* to parents or caregivers of young children. It's not always easy to talk about sex and sexuality with your children. Most parents don't get a lot of practice, so it's really important to be ready when the time comes. *From Birth to Puberty* offers a comprehensive, positive, easy to read guide that has been written from experience, expertise and understanding. I will be adding this book to the FPA Bookshop catalogue."

-Noelene Smith, National Resource and Health Promotion Manager,
New Zealand Family Planning Association.

From Birth to Puberty

helping your child develop
a healthy sexuality

Gill Lough and Max Saunders

SUNTIME
NAPIER

From Birth to Puberty has been written to help parents foster a healthy sexuality in their children. None of the suggestions or information is intended to replace the advice of health professionals. Neither the publisher nor the authors can accept responsibility for injuries or illness arising from a failure by a reader to take professional advice. Every effort has been made to trace copyright holders of quotes in this book. However, any error will gladly be corrected by the publisher for future printings.

Contents

Contents

At School

Special situations

Endnotes

Acknowledgements

Many people have contributed ideas and knowledge to this book. Our thanks go to parents, friends and educators for their willingness to share their personal stories with us informally and in workshops. Their frankness and generosity have helped to bring the book alive. Thanks to the New Zealand Family Planning Association for their positive approach to sexuality and for the learning opportunities that have shaped our thinking. Special thanks for their technical assistance to Ken Maclaren and Sally Woods.

We are indebted to our reviewers: Sonia Cunningham, Brenda Lewis, Carol Lough, Glenys Wood, Oliver Smales, Max Abbott, Fran Hagon, Tess Conran-Liew, Sue Bagshaw, Margaret Sparrow, Elaine Higham, Joan Plowman, Elizabeth Perales, Sue Doring, Jane Lennan.

About the authors

Gill Lough and Max Saunders have more than 20 years experience in adult, family and sexuality education, and qualifications in occupational therapy, paediatrics, science and education.

Gill Lough has 15 years experience in sexuality education with the New Zealand Family Planning Association. She works with parents, children, adolescents, teachers, health professionals and community workers. Max Saunders has 20 years experience in adult education, including senior lecturer in health science at Eastern Institute of Technology. They live in Hawke's Bay, New Zealand, and have 3 children.

Getting Started

1

Introduction

We love our children.

We think children are fantastic, and deserve the best possible start to life.

And since you have taken the time to pick up this book, we assume you do too.

This book is for people who want to learn about the development of children's sexuality, from birth to puberty. It is written especially for parents of young children. You have an important, challenging and very rewarding task ahead. This is your opportunity to gain the skills and knowledge to help your child develop a healthy sexuality.

Our sexuality is an integral part of who we are. For adults, a healthy sexuality means we feel good about ourselves, enjoy our sensuality and can openly express feelings of affection, love and intimacy. Our sexuality develops from birth and continues throughout our lives. But just mentioning children and sexuality in the same breath can make parents uncomfortable.

> *Danny has just turned two and Mia is still a baby. They are so pure and innocent I can't imagine them as teenagers. The thought of them having any kind of sexual development while they are children seems wrong to me. Surely it's too early to think about sexuality when the kids are so young.*
>
> -Helen, mother of two

Talking about children's sexuality can make us feel uneasy because we often assume that sexuality means the same for children as it does for adults. But child and adult sexuality are different in fundamental ways. Children's sexual behaviour does not have the same meaning and does not occur with the same thoughts and feelings as similar adult behaviour.

What is sexuality?

Sexuality is an integral part of the personality of everyone – man, woman and child. It is a basic human need and an aspect of being human that cannot be separated from other aspects of human life.

-World Health Organisation[1]

It is the energy that motivates us to find love and contact, feel warmth and intimacy. It is expressed in the way we feel, move and touch and are touched. It is about being sensual as well as sexual.

-University of Minnesota[2]

Sexuality includes all those things in our lives that relate to being a girl or boy, a man or a woman. For adults it can include sexual intercourse, but sexuality is far more than sex. It is a basic part of who we are and is reflected in our values, attitudes and behaviour. It influences the way we feel about other people. Our sexuality helps us show love, compassion, joy and sorrow. It includes our gender – the sexual differences between men and women that are determined socially rather than biologically - and shapes our personality. Sensuality is also an important part of sexuality. Sensuality is the way we appreciate the world through our senses - sound, sight, touch, taste, smell and movement.

Sexuality is affected by our biological makeup and our social and emotional development as we progress through childhood. Language, intellectual, physical and social skills develop in stages from birth through adulthood. Similarly, sexuality also develops in stages from birth.

> *I was helping at the pre-school and went to tidy up the playhouse area. I was shocked to find two four-year-olds lying in the bed together. They had no clothes on and were wriggling and giggling under the sheets. My first thought was they were acting out sex they had seen on TV or even at home.*
>
> –JoAnn, mother of a pre-schooler

The children in this story were enjoying the physical sensations of their skin against the sheets and each other. Their actions were playful, sensual and exciting, not filled with sexual desire, arousal or eroticism. JoAnn thought about this difference and recognised the child-like nature of their play. She was then able to relax, laugh with the children – and at her own reaction – and encourage them to hop out of bed and put their clothes on.

How would you have reacted if your child was involved? A lot of parents are surprised by the sexual nature of their child's play and are unsure what, if anything, they should do. Important issues like these arise from an early age and they need to be dealt with in a positive manner for your child to develop a healthy sexuality.

Guiding your child's sexuality

Guiding children's sexuality as they grow up is a challenge for all parents. Many parents succeed brilliantly and the information in *From Birth to Puberty* is based on the knowledge gained from studying, researching and working with families and with parenting and sexuality education organisations.

Helping your child develop a healthy sexuality is a process that takes many years – a whole childhood – so you have time to learn and to develop your skills. *From Birth to Puberty* will help you prepare for the changes in sexuality that occur in the first 12 years, up to and including puberty. You can respond to your child's needs and questions involving sexuality as they arise. You can take the initiative and use everyday opportunities and incidents to talk to and teach them about sexuality. It then becomes a normal and comfortable part of their lives.

Different families

There are many different family combinations involved in parenting. Yours may be a family of mum, dad and two kids, or some other family group. You may be a parent, step-parent, relative or caregiver responsible for raising children. To avoid repeating these terms, throughout the book we have used the word *parent* to denote everyone in the role of parenting.

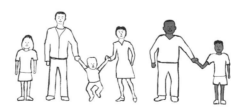

2

About this book

Why *From Birth to Puberty*?

Sexuality is a positive and core part of children's development. Many books on children's sexuality are either written for children or are for parents of 10 to 15-year-olds - the age parents traditionally begin to talk to their children about puberty and sex. Waiting until your child is ten before considering their sexuality is too late. We recommend that you think about your child's sexual development much earlier - from birth. We encourage you to foster communication from birth so that when your child reaches puberty you have established a comfortable two-way communication about sexuality.

Why start so young?

Some parents are surprised that we advise starting sexuality education so young. A typical comment:

Surely kids don't need to know about sex. They are too young and innocent.

That's true, very young children don't need to know about sex. However you can help your child if you are aware of the sexual development that is occurring. They do need to know their body is special, to know how to express their feelings, to feel good about being a girl or boy, and to be aware of the changes puberty will bring. These are aspects of their sexuality, as opposed to knowing about sex.

From Birth to Puberty is designed specifically for parents and others taking responsibility for children. It is not for children to read - there are other books written especially for children about sex. In fact most children today will have a better technical knowledge of sex than their parents did at the same age. Our emphasis is on sexuality not sex. Sex education is about the biological facts. Sexuality education is more holistic and includes family and lifestyle issues.

However, from our experience of teaching and working with young people we believe children need to start learning about sex well before they reach adolescence. Young children are engaging in sexual activity or are under pressure to do so without an understanding of the physical, emotional or ethical implications.

Using this book

From Birth to Puberty is organised into 5 parts:

- *Getting started* – describes the differences between child and adult sexuality, and takes you through a typical parent workshop on children's sexuality.

- *Children's sexual development* - follows sexual development from birth to puberty and suggests ways of responding to the issues that arise.

- *Ask me anything* – shows you how to communicate openly about sexuality with your child and respond confidently to their questions. How values and attitudes affect sexuality and ways you can foster positive values and attitudes in your child.

- *At school* - outlines sexuality education at primary school, addressing questions and concerns you may have with the school teaching sexuality to your child. Explains how you can have input into your school's sexuality education program and includes examples of the content of a typical primary school program.

- *Special situations* - looks at specific sexuality issues for single parents and stepfamilies, and at keeping your child safe from sexual abuse and underage sex.

Reading *From Birth to Puberty* will give you knowledge about children's sexuality. Actually using that knowledge to help your child, by converting the knowledge into action, is the difficult part. Knowing what to do is not enough: you need to know *how* to do what needs to be done. Throughout the book are suggestions and exercises to show you how. At the end of each chapter in *Children's sexual development* are activities specifically for each age. Make notes of what you have tried, and ideas that you would like to try. Working through the exercises will help you interact positively with your child about sexuality issues.

Stories and quotes

Reading other parents' stories helped me to see ways I could talk to Teela-Jay about the changes she was about to go through. I was surprised when she told me she had been waiting for me to tell her about periods. Her friends had been talking and when they saw she didn't know about periods they said, "You'll have to wait 'til your mother tells you".

-Natasha, mother of Teela-Jay, 8 years

Sharing stories from children and parents gives you an insight into how other parents have dealt with situations in their own families. Where we have quoted them directly we have changed their names to protect their privacy. We don't have all the answers and there isn't one right way to respond to an incident or behaviour. Hearing what other parents have said and done will help you decide on your own personal approach. The theories that have contributed to our thinking remain in the background. The stories and practical activities will encourage you to approach your child's developing sexuality with confidence.

Why we wrote this book

Writing *From Birth to Puberty* arose directly from the experience of running workshops for parents of young children. Parents requested information or a book written for parents on children's sexuality. We found there was no single book that covered all the material parents wanted. We also have professional concerns over some aspects of children's sexual experimentation at puberty, and believe parent education and awareness about young children's sexuality can limit this behaviour.

We live in New Zealand, surrounded by the vast oceans of the South Pacific. Despite this isolation, our young children are exposed to messages about sex through media: on TV, video, through music lyrics, movies, magazines and the Internet. Many of the messages and images are of concern to parents or are inappropriate for the age of the child. Parents around the world face a similar challenge - how to help their children develop a healthy sexuality in an environment of increasing exposure to media messages about sex.

What fresh insights into child sexuality can we give from this part of the world? First, a diverse cultural perspective, with examples from Maori and Pacific Island parents as well as European New Zealanders. Second, New Zealand has a progressive primary school health and sexuality education curriculum, in which parent input is encouraged. We are promoting a collaborative approach between parents and teachers to deliver a holistic sexuality program from the time your child starts school. And finally, we have our own professional experience gained in 20 years of adult, family and sexuality education.

3

Children's sexuality

Two five-year-old boys are being chauffeured to a party. One says to the other: "I had a dream I was sexing with a girl." Giggles and snorts cocoon them until the other thinks of a comeback that goes one better. "Well ...I had a dream I was sexing with Robert."

Big ears at the wheel is riveted. Has my son just come out? ... These boys in short pants all have their baby teeth, yet already they are talking about losing their virginity.

But then I remember getting engaged to Roderick Davis in kindergarten and scenes behind the shelter shed and soon I'm more relaxed about the fact that sexuality is more exotic these days...

-Kate Legge[3]

Some of these thoughts may go through your mind as you try to understand incidents involving your child's sexuality. Young children talking about sex can make us uncomfortable. Children are perceived as innocent, while sex is not. However the images and information about sex that young children are now exposed to means they use language and know more of the facts of sex than children even a decade ago. But children's language and sexual behaviour does not have the same meaning as it does for adults.

Differences between child and adult sexuality

Mary felt very uncomfortable when her five-year-old son Matt pressed his groin into her thigh as she lay on the couch. When he leaned over and began to play with her breast she thought he had gone beyond curiosity. She felt very confused.

Like Mary, you may have concerns about whether your child's sexual behaviour is normal. In many cases this concern is unfounded and is due to misunderstanding how child sexuality differs from adult sexuality. Parents sometimes attribute adult meanings to children's behaviour. You may see similarities between the sexual behaviour of children and adults, and mistakenly think they have the same motives. For instance when your five-year-old hugs, kisses and sensually touches you, it may seem that there is an erotic component to their behaviour. However it is much more likely that it is just a demonstration of affection for you.

Children's play involving sex or sexual roles is universal. Incidents such as a four-year-old boy lying on top of his fully clothed mother and saying "I want to make love to you" is likely to be mimicking something they have seen on TV. Your three-year-old touching your genitals is most likely to be harmless curiosity on their part. They may also be testing boundaries, to see where you set limits. Their language and behaviour may appear adult-like but it lacks the passionate, erotic component of adult sexuality. Bernie Zilbergeld tells a story about a son wanting to have a penis as big as his father. When his father asked why he said, "So I'll be able to pee more, silly"[4].

When adults talk about 'having sex' they are usually referring to sexual intercourse. And when adults talk about 'sex' the word can include a range of sexual activity including kissing, caressing, fondling, oral or genital sex. President Clinton's impeachment proceedings highlighted the debate over the definition of sex, but for adults the word sex is associated with sexual feelings, arousal and excitement. Young children don't have the same knowledge or experience. Even if they have seen sex on TV or other media their ideas are limited to thinking 'sex' is kissing or rubbing around together. They don't understand the concept of feeling sexy or 'turned on'.

> *At lunchtime a group of 7-year-olds were playing in the school playground. Two boys were waiting in the centre of the 'tunnels', concrete pipes placed at angles for the children to crawl through. The girls dared each other to crawl in to meet the boys, where they would receive a kiss. The kiss was a quick peck on the cheek. One girl thought this was very naughty and went to tell the teacher. "Miss, the boys are sexing the girls in the tunnels".*

As in this story, children's sexual play is normal if it involves curiosity and play; if it is spontaneous and open; and if it involves sensuality and excitement, rather than eroticism. Young children have low levels of the hormone testosterone, which is required for erotic feelings. Testosterone levels rise at adolescence, so young children do not experience the sexual desire that adolescents and adults do.

Children's innocence

A concern you may have is that giving your child the facts about sex will take away their innocence, the qualities of wonder and naivety children have. Researchers argue against this however, pointing out that children's understanding is limited regardless of how much information they are given.[5] There is a large gap between child and adult reasoning and comprehension. This gap protects young children's innocence. Although you give them information on sex and sexual matters, they do not understand or act on it in the way adults do.

Encouraging your child's feelings of comfort about sexuality and discussing sexual matters is what you want to achieve. However you will also want to set boundaries for your child's sexual expression and behaviour. To achieve both these goals requires a balance between the two. For example, if you are the mother of a five-year-old who repeatedly touches your breasts, you can say, "I don't want you touching my breasts, my breasts are private". This sets a boundary, and your child learns it is your personal space.

Setting this limit prevents your child's innocent curiosity from developing into problem behaviour. Say it in a light-hearted way. This will keep your child comfortable. A balance is then achieved between comfort and setting limits. Setting too many limits may make your child anxious and uncomfortable talking about sexuality.

Messages

Parents have a significant influence on their child's sexuality. Throughout *From Birth to Puberty* the term 'messages' is used to convey the idea that what we say and how we say it reflects our values and attitudes about sexuality. You give both verbal and nonverbal messages from what you say and by your behaviour. Your child will observe the way you relate to others and how you express love and affection. Your cultural background also influences the sexuality messages you convey.

What you don't say also communicates your values and attitudes. Even when you do not respond verbally your facial expression or other body language can give a strong message. How you communicate helps form your child's attitude toward sexuality. They learn as much or more from your emotional reactions as they do from what you actually say. Your child also gets messages about sexuality from their friends, from television, movies, advertising, in song lyrics and other media. However your messages are the most important, especially in the early years.

We believe that it is important for you as parents to talk together about the messages you plan to give your child. If you are a single parent you could talk with another adult to help clarify your ideas and values. For example, talk about the words you will teach your child for the sexual parts of the body. Deciding ahead of time on the underlying messages you want to give will make it easier to raise issues with your child and response to their questions. You will also say what you really meant to say and not give some other message.

Messages from the media

Children are exposed to sexual messages from the media, especially on TV, from the time they are toddlers. Producers of programs and commercials use sex to gain viewer attention, knowing it will increase their market share of the available audience. Daytime and early evening TV shows that young children watch from age two can have sexual imagery and unrealistic portrayals of sexual themes. You will have to make decisions at an early age about what your child views, and how much exposure they have to movies, TV talk shows and other programming that has sexual content.

Pre-teens or *tweens* - girls aged eight to 12 - are targeted by magazines using the sexualization of young girls to promote cosmetics, clothing and pop music. Marketers call it 'kargoy' – Kids Are Getting Older Younger. What used to appeal to 12-year-olds can now be made appealing to 8-year-olds.

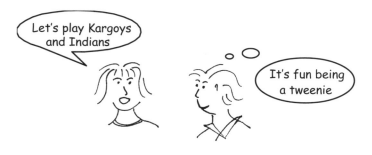

Take a look at magazines whose readership are girls of six to ten years, judging by the reader's letters and photographs. They use pre-teen models in suggestive outfits and plenty of makeup to sell fashion and other products. Lipstick advertisements picture pre-teen madeup models: "Lavish your lips with Liquid Lips…Kiss Kiss!" and a naked teenage girl with the words: "When everything else comes off, Lipcote stays on".

Here is an example quote from a reader's letters page:

> Reader: *I'm nine and I think a boy in my class likes me but I don't really know if he does or not. Please help me.*
>
> Magazine: *Wow! It sounds like you like him, and how unreal that he might like you too!? The best thing is to treat him like a friend and see how well you get on. Then who knows what will happen? You might start a little relationship! Go girl!*[6]

Pre-teen girls are also reading magazines aimed at teenagers that contain explicit sex messages and advice. Features such as '*What's your flirting style?*', '*When it's time to make a move on your crush*', '*How to be a better lover*', are standard fare in teen mags, and are readily available to younger girls. Parents of pre-teens are often unaware of the material in their daughter's magazines.

> *I buy that magazine for my 8-year-old daughter every week. I've never looked at it!*
>
> -Macy, mother of two

When mothers take a closer look at the content they are often surprised. They feel angry at the pressure put on their children to be sexually attractive before they have reached puberty.

Sexual messages in the media influence your child's attitudes and behaviour. Pre-teens do not have a well-developed ability to judge media critically, and are easily influenced by these images and information. Some of the messages on TV and other media about sexuality are positive. Many magazines for pre-teens do give practical responsible advice, and do address their anxieties and the issues that are most important to them at that age. There are some very responsible TV programs that show adults or teenagers in healthy relationships, and handling relationship problems in positive ways. There are many others that portray unrealistic or compulsive sexual behaviour, such as two people meeting for the first time and leaping into bed ten minutes later. Soap operas show attractive people having regular affairs, or using sex to escape their daily problems.

For young people, Internet chat rooms are exciting but can be addictive. Kids meet their peers and can form online attachments with them. There is a risk of your child meeting sexual predators in chat rooms and sending their phone number, address or picture to these adults, who may pose as young people. In teen chat rooms that pre-teens can join, sex is a hot topic, and personal information, fantasies and desires are exchanged.

Sex in the media is here to stay. You can monitor what your child is watching on TV, what they are reading and the time they spend on the net. As you develop family rules about reading, TV viewing, joining Internet chat rooms and using other media, you will be giving positive messages to your child about your own values.

4

Ask yourself this

Ask yourself this question:

How old do I want my child to be when they have their first kiss?

10?… 13?… 18?… Or maybe 21 or 25?
Okay, so 25 is unrealistic. Try 13.

What skills and personal qualities do I want them to have by then?

To be playful, fun-loving, sensual and affectionate? To be the most popular girl in the class? To be a sensitive new-age guy or a macho, manly stud? To be a straight talker, confident and assertive? To feel strong, to value themselves and know where they are going? To be streetwise and sexwise? To have a karate black belt?
Okay, fine. Now think,

What was I like when I had my first kiss? Had my parents taught me all I needed to know by then?

Probably not.
You learned some things about sexuality from your parents, but you also learned from your friends, your own explorations and

experiences, from books, magazines, TV, videos, religious groups, school, and others in your family. And there was probably a lot you didn't know.

A parent workshop

The series of questions we have just put to you are typical of those asked at the beginning of parent workshops on children's sexuality. Apart from you participating in the workshop, the next best thing we can do is to take you through the first part of a typical sexuality workshop for parents of young children.[7]

Parents are asked:

> *How old do you want your child to be when they have their first kiss?*

Usually parents joke that they would like their child to be over 20 years old, fully mature physically and emotionally knowing everything they need to know before they enter a sexual relationship.

Parents are then asked to think how well prepared they were when they had their first kiss with sexual feelings. The parents think about this to themselves – they don't share their thoughts with others. Parents reflect on their own learning when they were children, and the role their own parents had in their sexuality education.

This statement is put to the group:

> *My parents were the primary source of information about sexuality for me.*

Parents are then asked to stand along a line on the floor of the room, with those who strongly agree with the statement at one end, to those who strongly disagree at the other end, and others at points in-between. Most parents place themselves at or near the strongly disagree end. They are then invited to comment.

Typical comments are:

> *In our family we weren't allowed to mention sex at all. You soon learned not to ask questions, because you were sent out of the room.*

> *My father was a single parent. When I was 12 he told my older sister to pass on to me a book he had given her about sex. He said, "Tell him to read this". I read it but I didn't ever talk to Dad about it. He never mentioned it. I think he just didn't know how to bring up the subject, or was too embarrassed. A couple of weeks later my sister took the book away and I never saw it again.*

> *We had sex education at high school. It was all about sperm and fallopian tubes, not about relationships. Nothing at primary school that I can remember or from my parents.*

> *My parents were very open and talked to us. My mum is still the person I go to to talk about anything.*

The discussion brings out how parents did learn about sex: from books "in the library, hoping no one was watching", from personal experience and experimentation, talking to brothers, sisters, friends. Some of the comments such as "Sex was never mentioned" are unfair to our parents however. Remember that learning about sexuality is more than talking about sex. You learned about relationships and the expression of feelings from your parents. You learned the behaviour expected of a boy or girl and respect for others. You learned communication skills, relationship skills and how to care for yourself and others.

Sources of information for my child

Parents are then asked to take their places on a line, again from strongly agree to strongly disagree with the statement:

I am the primary source of information about sexuality for my child right now.

This time parents tend to be more evenly spread along the line. Again parents are invited to comment.

Yes, because my child is only 2, and I wouldn't want it any other way.

My Johnny is 10, and he comes to me when he wants to know anything and I don't think he'd go anywhere else to ask it.

They probably are influenced by other people. My kids are 5 and 7, and they make new friends easily and go to other people's homes. I hear the stories the kids bring home.

There is a range of opinion expressed. Parents who strongly agree are often surprised at the comments by others along the line. From listening to these comments they begin to realise that they will not be the only sources of their young child's learning about sexuality. They see that their child will have many outside influences on their learning, especially once they start pre-school and primary school. Many parents say they find it a bit scary that they won't be able to protect their children from other influences. They can't imagine what they will be like as teenagers and are often horrified at the thought that their young children could then begin sexual relationships.

How can I stop her becoming a teenager – I want Michelle to stay my baby!

What will they be like as an adult?

Let's look at the question again. What are the personal skills and qualities you would like your children to have by the time they begin relationships with sexual attraction and sexual feelings? Remember you are preparing your child now so that when the time comes they will have the confidence to enjoy this exciting new stage in their lives. Here are some typical responses from parents at parenting workshops:

They will have a healthy respect for themselves and others.

They will feel good about who they are and feel positive about themselves physically.

They will have a sense of humour and enjoy relaxing and having fun.

They will be able to express their feelings both emotionally and verbally.

They will be good listeners and clearly express what they want.

They will be able to negotiate and approach making decisions with confidence.

These are great answers and show exactly the skills children need. With these skills your child will be developing a strong foundation about who they are and what they want. Your values will guide them as they learn from others. When things go wrong they will have the resources to keep their head above water. And you will be able to take most of the credit.

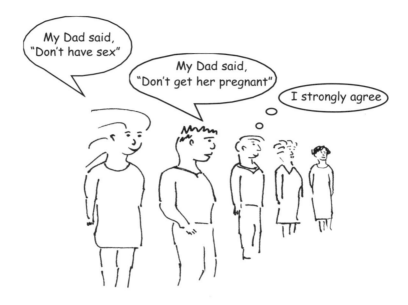

Why learn about children's sexuality?

Why set yourself the task of understanding the sexual development of your child from birth to puberty? Did your parents understand their influence on your sexual development when you were a baby? Chances are they didn't think about it much. Here is a summary of the reasons we think you should take on this responsibility.

BECAUSE PARENTS ARE FIRST TEACHERS

You are the first and most important source of learning about sexuality for your child. You begin your sexuality teaching when they are a baby, and it continues through their childhood and teenage years. The emotional bond you form with your baby is their first experience of a gentle, warm, loving relationship. You naturally show your love by kissing, cuddling and caressing them. As your child grows they will imitate you and learn to show affection in return.

Young children learn about their sexuality through their play and their curiosity. It won't be until reaching puberty that your child will become aware of sexual feelings and sexual attractions. By this time you will have helped them gain the skills they need to care for themselves. You will also have helped them develop a strong set of values so they can make healthy decisions in their lives.

TO IMPROVE YOUR PARENTING SKILLS

Guiding a child's learning about sexuality involves many different parenting skills. To do it well requires an understanding of the physical and emotional development of children from birth through adolescence. It requires the ability to have open and honest conversations without embarrassment. It helps if you are clear about your own values and attitudes toward sexuality and are willing to talk about them with your partner or other adults. You can then confidently share your family values with your child.

A positive outcome of practicing these parenting skills is that it will not be necessary to have 'The Big Talk' about sex with your child as they start puberty. Of course you will be talking to your child about sex at that age but it will not be a special one-off talk or series of talks. You will already have had healthy two-way communication with your child for many years. The combination of understanding your child's sexual development from birth, developing open and honest communication, and expressing your values will enhance your relationship with them and prepare them for their teenage years.

FOR YOUR CHILD'S COMFORT

You can foster your child's feelings of comfort about sexuality and their ability to discuss sexual matters. As a parent you have a significant and lasting influence on your child's sexuality. Children deserve to feel confident and enjoy their sexuality. Give them positive messages about sexuality so they go on to be confident, loving, caring adults and form positive relationships.

TO COUNTER SEXUAL MESSAGES IN THE MEDIA

The environment for children has changed from a generation ago. Children today get more information about sex from more sources: TV, movies, the Internet, in advertising across all media. And the sexual imagery is more explicit. Marketers use sexualized images of pre-teens in magazines to sell products to young girls that were once aimed at teenagers. To balance the unreal portrayal of sex and sexual relationships that most children have seen on TV and in other media by the time they are seven you need to talk about your own values and explain what you believe and why.

TO SET BOUNDARIES

Many parents feel that by introducing these issues they will destroy their child's innocence. Boundaries are family rules for touching, speaking and behaving. Setting boundaries for sexual expression will help you preserve your child's innocence. An innocent child is inoffensive, free of guilt and naïve about sexual matters. Inappropriate boundaries or no limits to your child's sexual behaviour may lead to them losing their innocence. They may disregard other people's personal space or privacy, or harass them.

FOR YOUR CHILD

You want your child to grow up healthy, to have committed, loving relationships and lasting friendships. You want them to have values and attitudes that will enable them to survive and thrive and lead a fulfilling life. You want them to gain independence and good decision-making skills. Central to achieving all of these is the development of a healthy sexuality.

Children's Sexual Development

Children's sexual development

This part of *From Birth to Puberty* describes the sexual development of children and the influence parents have on their development. We have divided the time from birth to puberty into five general stages: babies, toddlers, pre-schoolers, primary school children and puberty.

The following table shows the age ranges for the five stages. The age range is a general guide only. For example, some boys will not have started puberty by the time they are twelve. Children develop at different rates and there are many influences that hinder or hasten their development.

Chapter	Stage	Age range
5	Babies	0 - 18 months
6	Toddlers	1 - 3 years
7	Pre-schoolers	3 - 5 years
8	Primary school	5 - 9 years
9 & 10	Puberty	9 - 12 years

Reading through these chapters you will find that the same issues are revisited, for example, setting boundaries, rules, learning about gender. We have done this so that the issues are addressed in an appropriate way as they arise in each stage of your child's development.

5

Babies

Zac is 3 months old. He snuggles into his mother's breast, feeling her warmth and softness against his cheek. His tongue plays with her nipple and he tastes the last sweet drops of her milk. The rhythm of her breathing, her smell and her smile are familiar. He gazes into her eyes and quietly watches her smile down at him. He yawns and stretches. Feeling well satisfied and relaxed, he drifts off to sleep.

At birth, babies can see and hear; touch and taste; cry, feed, and move their limbs. Their brain is receiving, processing and responding to all this sensory information. Zac's sexuality is forming on the foundation of these early sensory and social experiences.

You may think that there is not much sexual development occurring during the first 12 months of life. It is true there are far more obvious periods of sexual development in later childhood. And with the sleepless nights and constant care and attention the baby needs, most parents will be relieved just to get through this period. However the first 12 months are a period of rapid learning. Newborn babies enter the world with their parent's genetic mixture and experiences from the womb already shaping their development and behaviour.

Child development studies show that language, physical, social and intellectual development occurs in stages from infancy to adulthood. Sexuality follows a similar path. Knowing what to expect at a certain age helps you understand that a behaviour of concern to you may be typical at that stage of your child's sexual development.

Sexual development is one area of your baby's development. Other areas influence children's sexual development, including hearing and speech (talking), social and emotional development (expressing feelings, relating to others), sensory perception (vision, touch, smell, and taste), and physical skills (playing games). These all overlap and interact in the sexual development of your growing child.

The first 12 months

Babies hear sounds while in the womb and associate the sound of their mother's voice with comfort and warmth. After birth they respond to her voice by becoming quiet as she approaches and turning toward the sound of her voice. They focus on their mother's face and start smiling at about two months old. You learn to recognise the different cries your baby has when they are uncomfortable, lonely or hungry.

When your baby starts rolling and moving around on their stomach they also become more responsive to others in the family by laughing and babbling. From 6 months of age they begin to be suspicious of strangers. Gradually a sense of self develops and a concept that they are separate from others around them.

By the time they take their first steps they show a wide range of emotion such as sadness, affection, joy, fear, and annoyance. They will develop an emotional bond with one or more people. They will seek their attention, enjoy interacting with them, become distressed when separated from them and seek contact with them when unsure of a new situation.[1]

To some extent the sex of your baby will determine how you and others will treat them. Studies have shown we respond to baby boys and girls differently from birth, so that the baby is already learning the behaviours we expect from them as a boy or girl. How we talk, hold, dress, or play with them is different. Fathers tend to talk robustly with their sons, while mothers talk gently with their daughters. This sends subtle messages about the different expectations we have of girls and boys and begins the process of socialisation.

Babies are very sensual and experience pleasure from touching their genitals (penis or vulva) and will play with themselves when their nappies are off. Just as they learn that they have fingers and toes, they learn they have a penis or vulva.

Children have sexual sensations from birth. Baby boys have erections and baby girls secrete vaginal fluids. Smegma is a white waxy substance secreted by glands under the foreskin in boys and at the base of the labia in girls. Usually it will be washed away when you bathe the baby. However if it remains, bacterial action may cause an unpleasant smell.

The hormones in the mother's bloodstream sometimes cause the vulva of newborn girls to be enlarged. The same enlargement may occur in the breasts of both boys and girls at birth. Milk may even be produced. This settles down after a few weeks. Girls are born with ovaries full of egg cells which will develop throughout the reproductive part of their lives.[2]

I felt almost shocked by the size of my daughter's private parts when she was born. Nobody said anything but I was so relieved when she didn't look so out of proportion after a few weeks.

-Nancy, mother of three

Circumcision

Jane told this story at a parent workshop:

> *Jane's husband Bob, 40, was circumcised as a baby and had an expectation that his new son James would also have the operation. Bob was surprised when told by the doctor that the operation was no longer standard procedure and would not be performed at the unit where his son was born.*
>
> *Bob arranged for the operation with a surgeon at another facility. He was happy the operation had taken place. Little did he know that most of the foreskin was left intact. The surgeon had deliberately intended this as he believed the operation was unnecessary. Bob was happy in his ignorance, as Jane had never told him, and he had never taken a close look.*

Circumcision is the complete or partial removal of the foreskin of the penis. The operation is usually performed a few days after birth. When your first son is born you may not have given much thought to a decision about circumcision. You may feel pressured into making a hasty decision. You may feel that you have little choice as circumcision is not a routine procedure in many hospitals.

The foreskin is usually attached to the glans of the penis when the baby is born. It shouldn't be pulled back as it can cause tearing underneath. Most boys foreskin's can be pulled back by the time they are 3 or 4 years old, but this isn't necessary to clean the penis.

More about circumcision

In the operation the foreskin is cut to allow it to be pulled back behind the glans (head) of the penis. The foreskin consists of a double layer of skin that, without circumcision, covers the glans. Until recently in Western countries the operation has been widely practiced as a hygienic procedure. In many hospitals it has been routinely performed on newborn boys. It is estimated that circumcision occurs in about one sixth of the world's population and is probably the oldest surgical operation, dating back some 6000 years to ancient Egypt. Overall, the medical value of circumcision may be highest in places or countries where poverty and disease make good standards of hygiene difficult.

Parents may request circumcision for religious reasons. For traditional Jewish and Muslim families, circumcision is a religious duty, usually done shortly after birth or sometimes in childhood. In other cultures circumcision is part of a ritual performed at puberty, representing the end of childhood and the beginning of manhood. Other reasons people ask for their boys to be circumcised are because they believe circumcision will prevent disease, reduce masturbation, reduce sexual desire, as a treatment for bed-wetting or is necessary because the foreskin is too long.

The operation is now performed in Australia, New Zealand and the United Kingdom only if it is in the interests of the child, not the parents. As in other areas of medicine the trend is to avoid unnecessary intervention. The main medical reason to circumcise is when the foreskin prevents the normal flow of urine.[3]

Ann thought it was necessary to retract her 18-month-old son Johnny's foreskin to clean his penis. She was alarmed when she couldn't pull it back into position. Johnny became distressed when the end of his penis began to swell. Ann took Johnny to her family doctor who was also unable to reposition the foreskin. He was taken to a hospital where Johnny had to have an incision to ease the foreskin back. This meant that at a later date he had to have a partial circumcision.

This story highlights the risk of retracting the foreskin and not being able to return it. If this occurs take your son to see a doctor urgently.

Showing love and affection

Hugging, stroking and cuddling are very important to a baby's sexual development. Your baby learns how it feels to be loved when you cuddle them, talk softly and kiss them. This is how they learn to show love and affection when they are older. Some babies enjoy being kissed and cuddled. Others resist affection by arching back and pushing away.

Stella and her 20-something daughter Fiona were looking through the family photo albums. They noticed that the baby photos of Fiona's brother showed him looking relaxed and cuddly. But the baby photos of Fiona showed her holding her back bolt upright and arching away, no matter who was holding her. Stella recalled looking at Fiona when she was a baby and thinking, "You're a prickly little baggage aren't you".

This behaviour doesn't mean the baby doesn't like the person cuddling them. They are more likely to be very sensitive and reacting to too much handling. It's easy to see how this could influence the way you and others respond to your baby. If you perceive a negative response you will give them less attention. However the baby still needs the attention but not the cuddling.

Snuggling and caressing a baby is natural for most mothers but some fathers feel less comfortable doing this.

> *Simon felt uneasy about touching, cuddling or holding his baby daughter because of fears about what others would think. Could he be accused of sexual abuse? He felt it was such a grey area he withheld these normal affections from his baby.*

How could Simon distinguish between normal touching and sexual abuse? Normal touch is when touching is part of caring for the child. It is not normal when adults touch babies for their own sexual pleasure. Normal caring touch includes washing, drying and putting cream on the genital area. However even very young children can be taught to put cream on themselves.

Struggling to cope

Having a baby is supposed to be a wonderful experience but for many first time parents the 24 hour commitment comes as a bit of a shock. Sexuality development will be the last thing on your mind if you are struggling to cope with sleepless nights, constant crying and the endless cycle of feeding and cleaning up afterwards. Luckily in the first 12 months your child's sexuality will develop naturally. This is because of the love and affection you give your baby as you meet their demands for attention. You may already be enjoying some of the following activities with your baby.

Try these with your baby

- Massage your baby – learn through a book, video or go to a baby massage class.
- Allow your baby time to lie naked after a bath to get to know their body and feel the sensations of different surfaces such as a sheepskin, a silk sheet or your own body.
- Stimulate your baby with a feather, blow with a straw, shower them with bubbles or pour water gently all over their body in the bath.
- Practise using the 'proper' words for the sexual parts of the body as you tend to your baby so that you become comfortable saying them.

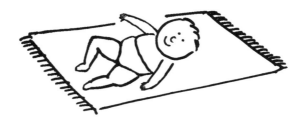

6

Toddlers

Zac squeals with delight as his mother pours water all over him as he lies wriggling in the bath. He slides up and down sloshing and tumbling in the waves he is making. He squeezes the soap, sending it like a missile into the air. His mother scoops him out and wraps him in a towel. Still wriggling and giggling, he is enjoying the wonderful sensations he is experiencing all over his body.

This squealing bundle of energy is now 12 months old. Soon he will be walking, climbing and running stiffly, swaying from side to side. He will develop the ability to pick up small toys and stack a few blocks.

As well as walking and other physical activity, toddlers can now feed themselves and show likes and dislikes of certain foods. Simple instructions are followed and they may use up to fifty words of their own. They describe what they are doing in simple sentences while they are busy playing. When they need to go to the toilet they tell someone. They show an interest in the physical difference between the sexes and learn to name the parts of the body. They recognise their reflection in a mirror.[4]

Independent little people

Their new independence extends to wanting to get their own way and they may have tantrums. They may become possessive with their toys. Toddlers like to play in the company of others but haven't learnt how to play interactive games with others. They become aware that their own actions can have an emotional impact on others and start to realise how other people may be feeling.

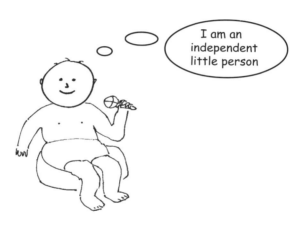

Toddlers begin to develop a concept that they are independent little people and not an extension of their mother or father. They continue learning about their bodies and play with their penis or vulva. They may also want to touch the sexual parts of their parent's body, to see what it feels like.

Murray liked to give his baby Jeremy a bath when he was having a bath himself. Jeremy loved it and they both had fun splashing and playing with Jeremy's toys in the water. When Jeremy was about 12 months he started to poke at Murray's penis. Murray laughed and told him not to do it. It became a game and one day Murray had an erection. Murray always made excuses to bathe separately after that. We didn't ever talk about it but I thought he must have thought it was weird to have happened with his kid. I didn't think anything of it really.

- Edith, Murray's wife

You may want to begin to set limits on your child touching your genitals but be mindful that they want to touch out of curiosity, not as an adult might for their sexual pleasure.

Learning about gender

Toddlers may not understand that their body parts are a permanent part of them. Young boys may worry that they might lose their penis when they see that girls don't have one, or girls may worry because they do not have a penis. You can help your child learn about the differences between a girl and a boy and encourage them to be positive about their gender. For example, if your daughter is concerned that she doesn't have a penis like her brother you could say, "You are a girl and have a vulva like Mummy and Johnny is a boy and has a penis like Daddy".

Touching their genitals

Sarah wondered if Tina, her 3-year-old daughter, was normal when she noticed that whenever she watched television she would stimulate herself by riding on the arm of the armchair. After sharing this with a parent group several other parents said they had noticed their daughters doing the same thing and that they had stopped doing it by the time they started school. Sarah felt quite relieved.

By the age of one most children enjoy touching their genitals. There are a number of reasons why your toddler may do this. It can be a way of finding out about their body and because it feels good. Toddlers may touch their genitals because they want to go to the toilet. They may touch their genitals because it gives them a feeling of comfort when they are worried.

Some children masturbate often. Little girls may rub themselves with a soft toy or ride on the arm of an armchair or rocking horse. Occasionally toddlers have been observed to have what appear to be orgasms. However masturbation at this age is usually a sensual, relaxing, comforting activity and not involving the intensity of sexual arousal and orgasm.

Some little boys constantly hold on to their penis. If the behaviour is concerning you, try to find out why they are doing it. It could be that something is worrying them. Very young children won't be able to tell you exactly what the problem is so you need to think about what could be the cause. It could be the new baby in the family, a parent going back to work or the scary dog next door. Work out how to help them feel better. Knowing you understand how they feel can be a great comfort to them. Alternatively it could be that they are rubbing themselves because they are itchy and may have eczema or an infection. It can simply be because they enjoy it and it has become a habit.

Setting boundaries

When you react to your toddler touching their genitals, think about the messages you want them to hear. You want them to know that their body is special but also private. By the time they are three years old they are able to learn that touching the sexual parts of their body is private, and not something people do in front of others.

Many mothers enjoy the intimacy of breast-feeding their babies. By the time their babies are toddlers they are usually weaned.

However some of the behaviours learned during this time may persist as this story indicates.

> *When Averil was breast-feeding Katherine, Katherine would tuck her hand inside her mother's blouse and onto her mother's breast. At 12 months when Averil carried her in her arms Katherine would still do the same, and place her hand on her breast. It became a habit and occurred particularly when Katherine needed reassurance or felt unsure of a situation. It started to become embarrassing for Averil as Katherine grew older.*

This was a difficult behaviour for Averil to change, and Katherine was not free of the habit until she was 2 and a half years old. Often we do not recognise that a behaviour has become a habit until it becomes a problem. We tell ourselves it's a stage they are going through and it will pass. When should you start setting boundaries to stop a behaviour becoming a habit? The best time is when you first start wondering if it could be a problem. Talking about it with a friend will put it in perspective and help you decide what to do.

> *When Darryn was 3 years old he liked to lift up my top and stroke my pregnant tummy and press his cheek against it. After his little sister was born he still did it, and I thought it was harmless at first. But he continued to do it and I became increasingly uncomfortable. I tried to stop him but he kept trying to lift my top even when he was five.*
>
> -Cindy, mother of two

This behaviour may have been appropriate when Cindy was pregnant but it became an issue when it continued after the birth of her baby. Darryn was not respecting Cindy's personal boundaries. If Cindy had set clear boundaries after the baby was born the problem would not have developed. Cindy could have said to Darryn, "Do you like feeling the skin on Mummy's tummy? I didn't mind you touching my tummy to feel the baby inside but now our baby is born I don't want you to do it". Setting boundaries is a balancing act though. Too many limits may cause anxiety or guilty feelings about sexuality and lead to your child avoiding talking about it with you.

Toilet training

Children are usually able to recognise the signs that they need to have a bowel motion by the time they are 2 years old. When your toddler starts to show this awareness toilet training can begin. They will usually be aware they need to urinate by the time they are 2½ years. Toilet training may take months and it is normal for children to have occasional accidents over the next couple of years. When toilet training is encouraged by praise, positive reinforcement and they are not put under pressure, children feel confident and in control. If they are punished or made to feel guilty when 'accidents' inevitably occur, they may associate their genitals with dirtiness and shame.

Rules

By the time toddlers turn two they are developing a sense of right and wrong. They show a concern over breaking adult rules such as making a mess in the bathroom or toilet, or not washing their hands. They may blame a toy for a toileting 'accident'. After age two they will test rules by breaking them and waiting to see whether you uphold the rule. They are now able to control their behaviour, for instance putting off playing a game with you until after lunch because there will be more time then. Toddlers appear to decide if what they want to do is right or wrong by whether it will bring them pleasure or punishment. These are signs of your child's developing moral sense.

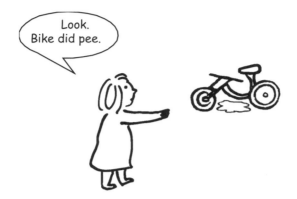

Discovered during sex

You may worry how to handle the situation when your toddler comes into your bedroom finding you making love. When a toddler observes their parents in a loving embrace they are unlikely to even notice that their parents are otherwise involved and are likely to demand attention for themselves. From the toddler's point of view you are preoccupied with each other and they want some of the attention.

Try these with your toddler

- Enjoy water play, using funnels, pipes, straws, tubing, containers, pieces of hose, ice cubes, bubbles and the garden sprinkler.
- Model gentle play with your toddler's toys and put words to the emotions they may feel if they were real. For example, if your child throws their teddy to the floor pick it up gently saying he looks sad and cuddle him "to make him better".
- If your toddler doesn't go to daycare create opportunities for them to be with other children of about the same age. They may find it hard to share toys so make sure there are enough toys or activities for all the children.
- Allow a time in the day to spend a quiet time together to maintain the intimate closeness you have had throughout your child's infancy.
- Play in front of the mirror and allow your toddler time to explore their mirror image.

7

Pre-schoolers

I was amazed at the difference in Lisa from age three to five. She was so active compared to her toddler days. Running, jumping, hopping, dancing, throwing and catching a ball, riding a tricycle. She could build structures with her blocks, cut things out with scissors, paint colourful pictures and draw with a crayon. She enjoyed imitating adults and liked to be helpful. She and her friends listened well to stories and they told long stories themselves. She played well with other kids. Her speech became fluent, she learned to count and she enjoyed jokes. She learned about the differences between girls and boys.

-Don, Lisa's father

Self identity

"I'm a girl like Mummy."

-Lisa, 3-year-old

By the age of 3 pre-schoolers will be able to tell you that they are a boy or a girl and will relate this to the parent of the same sex. If they have one or more siblings of the other sex they will know of the physical differences between the sexes. Pre-schoolers describe themselves in terms of their physical characteristics such as the colour of their hair and their size or in terms of their favourite activities.

They will not only identify as being male or female but also try to be like the people they are closest to. They will model their parent's behaviour and appearance and copy any expression of attitudes or prejudice by their parents.

> *I don't want to play with you 'cos my Dad says your Dad is gay.*
>
> -Lucy, 4-year-old

The oldest child in the family is likely to conform the most strongly to the values of their parents. If your child is from a minority culture they are more likely to be aware of cultural differences than children from majority cultures.

Emotionally, children at this age are becoming more independent. However they will continue to seek emotional support and physical closeness when they are anxious or stressed.

Favourite parents

> *When I grow up I'm gonna marry you Mummy.*
>
> -Tom, 4-year-old

Some pre-school children become intensely attached to the parent of the opposite sex and even feel jealous of the other parent. They want to snuggle up to them in bed, watch them get dressed and may want to touch their genitals. They may say that when they grow up they want to marry them. It is up to you to be understanding but also be honest. For example the favoured parent might say, "I love you too but when you grow up you will meet someone special to love". By the time they get to school this devotion to one parent will usually have become less intense.

Naming parts of the body

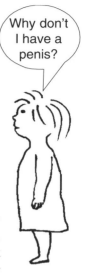

Why don't I have a penis?

Ben, a 7-year-old, was asked by his teacher how he could tell the difference between a girl and a boy. He replied, "A boy's got something sticking out like a hose".[5]

Ben wasn't sure what words to use. He used words like 'willy' or 'diddle' at home but didn't know what to say to his teacher at school. Children use language they are familiar with and if they haven't learnt the language that is commonly used they are confused. Learning to name the parts of the body is something most children do before they go to school. They need to know that it is acceptable to use words like penis and vulva or they may arrive at school with the belief that the correct words are dirty, rude or naughty. This creates a difficulty for teachers and parents when talking to children if they believe the correct words are offensive or forbidden. In the classroom the children may worry they will say the wrong thing.

Some people feel uncomfortable using the proper words for the sexual parts of the body. It is easier if you start using the anatomical words when your child is very young. There is nothing wrong with using other language at home, so don't be anxious if you don't want to use the correct terms. However if you do use baby names such as 'willy' for penis, your child still needs to know the anatomical names for all their body parts before they go to school. Pre-schoolers may be fascinated by a particular body part such as the navel and want to check if everyone else has one. You can show your pre-schooler picture books about their bodies and talk about how they work.

In the bathroom

Pre-schoolers are usually not modest about their bodies and like being naked. However children who observe adults being modest may start demanding privacy when dressing or using the bathroom. This behaviour is often inconsistent, as it is more about modelling adult behaviour than modesty. They become very interested in bathroom words and in what other people do in bathrooms and toilets. They are curious about the different positions men and women take when they use the toilet and will talk about it. For example, "Why do boys stand to pee?" Most girls will try to stand at least once when urinating.

When I was 5 years old I knew my brothers could stand to urinate so I decided to try myself. I tried to direct the stream into the toilet but it seemed to go everywhere. My mother accused my older brothers of the mess with such venom that I was too frightened to own up to it. My brothers were in trouble bigtime. We laughed about it later though.

-Stormee, young mother

Swearwords

"This is a fuckin' bucket." Jason said proudly holding his new bucket and spade high in the air.

-Jason, 4-year-old

Jason has the family's undivided attention. How will they react? Children learn swearwords if not from you, then from other children or adults. They become aware that these words are powerful and that they can get attention or a strong reaction from adults when they use them. Swearwords are often words to do with sex, or bottoms, or going to the toilet. These topics hold an intense interest for children because of the privacy and secrecy that surround them. Consequently children find there is something exciting and daring in using swearwords. They may create their own words such as *poo-face* or *widdle-diddle* and use them with delight.

How should you respond? Think about what you want your child to consider when using these words. You may want them to learn not to use that language at home, or that it is rude to swear or that it may upset other people when they hear them using these words. Children quickly learn that there are different rules for different places and situations. Sometimes it is simply best to ignore it. The fascination soon passes if they don't get a reaction.

Learning about gender

Pre-schoolers continue to learn about behaviours expected of boys and girls. Parents relate differently to their children depending on the child's gender. Girls usually take longer to develop an emotional independence from their parents. They tend to stay in a safe, secure environment and go back to their caregivers often for reassurance. Boys are usually more adventurous and have more confidence to explore their surroundings.

Children at 3 - 5 years in all societies are learning gender-related roles and relationships. They model their behaviour on the people they spend most of their time with and who they want to be like. They come to prefer the activities and roles that traditionally fit with the same-sex role stereotypes of their culture. Little girls like to play 'house' with their soft toys or dolls - making beds, cooking the dinner, doing the dishes, talking on the phone, dressing up to go to work and organising the household - if those are the roles she observes at home with her mother. Little boys also play 'house' in a similar way but tend to play more expansively, adding trucks and cars and building extra structures. Playing with soft toys and dolls is normal for both boys and girls. They are being caring and gentle, qualities usually seen as feminine but have equal value for men.

Boys and girls often select playmates of the same sex. Boys play in larger groups and their play is rougher and takes up more space.

Girls tend to form close relationships with one or two other girls. These friendships are marked by the sharing of thoughts, ideas and secrets.[6]

Both boys and girls like to dress-up as adults and may act out roles of the opposite sex. When a little boy puts on a dress and make-up it doesn't mean he is rejecting his male role. His activity does not have the same meaning it has for adult cross-dressers. When playing make-believe and dressing up as the opposite sex, children are spontaneously and openly acting out the various activities that are part of their everyday life. This is very different from the compulsion adult cross-dressers feel to dress as the opposite sex to express their sexuality, which is often in secret and characterised by guilt. In contrast the child is playing openly and having fun.

Sexual orientation refers to a person's feelings of sexual attraction to the same, the other or both sexes. Some parents worry that allowing their son to play games such as wearing a dress and make-up may influence his sexual orientation in later life. These parents' fears are groundless. Enjoying these feminine roles will not influence a boy's future sexual orientation. Comfort with being male or female (gender identity) is different from the sexual attraction people feel for each other (sexual orientation). Heterosexual men are comfortable with their male gender and so are homosexual men. Confusion about these issues and fear of homosexuality has caused many parents and other adults to limit how girls and boys express themselves in their play.[6]

Sex Play

William and Stacey had both recently turned 3 and were from different families. They lived in the same household and were always playing together. Stacey's mother Cherry walked into the bedroom to find William lying naked on the bed. Stacey was rubbing talcum powder all over his body. William was loving it and lay there with an erection. Cherry left them playing, feeling comfortable they were both enjoying themselves and that it was harmless play. 5 minutes later they were both busy playing outside.

Pre-schoolers start to become curious about the sexual differences between boys and girls, and compare themselves with others. They explore their bodies including their sexual parts. They learn by looking at each other, by touching and by playing games such as 'doctors and nurses' or mimicking adult sexual behaviour. Children's interest in sex and sex play does not take over their whole playtime and is just one of many things they want to explore.

Is your child's sex play normal? Parents often ask this. What is normal sexually oriented behaviour in 3 - 5 year-olds? A study found that children enjoyed being naked, and masturbated openly at age three, but less so by age five[7]. They found children's sex play, such as touching each other's genitals, involved curiosity rather than sexual awareness. Pre-schoolers are curious about their bodies and enjoy being touched. Young children love sensuality and seek physical experiences. Through play they learn lessons they will need to fully experience their sexuality as adults. Their play is characterised by excitement, sensuality, spontaneity and openness. It is easy for parents to forget that their child's sex play is very different from adult sexual activity, which is characterised by passion, eroticism and privacy.

As long as there is no physical danger, there is no need for parents to worry about sex play if the children are about the same age and size, and if the children are not being made to do something they don't want to do. When children are of a similar age and size it is less likely that one child will persuade the other to do something they are uncomfortable with. Most sex play is between children who are friends or siblings.

David shared this story at a parent's workshop:

I have three sons aged 4 to 7 who have lots of fun together. But they have a new game in the evening after their bath. They use the bed as a trampoline, jumping and rolling about naked. That's okay but they get very excited and have started grabbing each other's genitals. I'm wondering if I should stop them.

-David, father of three sons

After talking about the game with the other parents he decided the game could be unsafe and he would talk to his sons. The messages he wanted to give them was that their genitals were sensitive and easily hurt and they needed to be more careful in their play.

When children are found playing sex games they are often embarrassed, especially if they learn their parents do not approve. If they are asked to stop and play something else they will, at least while adults are present. They usually enjoy these games just as they do other games but they won't be particularly upset by changing activities.

If you find children playing sex games and you are not sure how to react, take a deep breath and think first. Many things children find confusing or frightening are caused by the way parents react. If you show dismay or indicate your child's behaviour is dangerous they may become concerned that something bad will happen to them. If they aren't worried or upset about the game, treat it in a low-key manner and redirect them if you think it is necessary. Think about the message you want to get across to your child. This message will be important in their developing understanding of sex and sexuality.

The message might be that it is okay to be curious about others but that the sexual parts of their own and others' bodies are private. You could say:

I see you are playing a game about your bodies. You can learn by looking at each other but remember that this part of your body is private. You can also learn by looking at books. Let's go and look at some books together.

Setting clear boundaries in a non-judgemental way will guide your child away from unsafe activities. For example, you may need to be clear that it isn't safe to push anything into the vagina (a common experiment during water play).

How are babies made?

A three-year-old cannot grasp the concept that babies are made or that time existed before they were born. They think that babies simply exist.[8] They don't usually understand or ask about sexual intercourse. However in the next few years they will develop some idea that babies are made by parents. They want to know where babies come from, how babies get into a mother's body and how they get out. If they ask how babies are made they need a simple answer. It is usually enough to say that the baby is made when the father puts a special seed into the mother's womb where it joins up with a tiny soft egg.

Your child will relate the terms you use to what they know. If you talk about a seed growing in Mummy's tummy they may imagine a plant growing in soil in her stomach. If you talk about eggs they usually think of a hen's egg, which has a brittle shell. If you notice your child is confused think about the words you have used. Asking

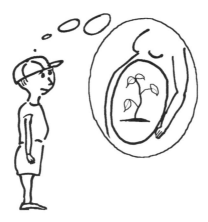

"Daddy planted a seed in Mummy's tummy"

them to tell you what they think will give you the chance to clear up any misunderstandings.

> How did the baby get into your tummy?

They may ask, "Did I grow in Mummy's tummy?" and "How did I get out?". Try to answer in simple language but use the correct words. "A special place in Mummy's tummy called the womb" or "When you were ready to be born the womb helped to push you through a stretchy opening called the vagina between Mummy's legs".

Both boys and girls have questions about their bodies. It is important to teach both boys and girls about the anatomy of both sexes and to explain that there's a special reason why their bodies are different. For more on answering your child's questions take a look at the *Ask me anything* section of this book.

Setting boundaries - public and private

Boys sometimes think it's exciting to look under a girl's dress. Both girls and boys think it is funny and exciting to watch children of the opposite sex going to the toilet. They often giggle and make jokes about bathrooms and toilets and about what people do in the bathroom or toilet. Once again you can explain to your child about the private parts of the body and that the bathroom is a private place. Explain the difference between public and private. You could say, "The private parts of the body are the parts we cover up when we go for a swim". Showing them pictures of the human body in picture books written for children will help them learn about sex differences. Through your example they also learn to treat the issue with more respect.

You may have set limits and tried to teach your child to respect their sexuality but a worrying behaviour persists. If your child keeps repeating a disturbing sexual behaviour, or if anger or excessive anxiety accompanies the behaviour you may need to discuss it with a health professional.

Discovered during sex

A group of women were sharing stories about their children and one mentioned that her four-year-old had charged into their bedroom while they were making love. "Thank God that's never happened to us!" said her friend.

Many parents agree. Why are they anxious? Apart from the embarrassment they are often concerned that their child will lose their innocence about sex. But children at this age only have a limited understanding of sex in spite of what they have seen you doing. In their eyes you are playing games or having fun together. In some cases they may think you are fighting or even hurting each other.

Gemma could hear her parents making noises and when she went to investigate could see her mother was getting squashed underneath her father. She tried to push him off saying, "Get off Mummy, you are hurting her".

Gemma's mother can give her reassurance that she isn't hurt and that they are having fun together. Respond to your child's presence in a natural way and they will not be concerned by what they have seen. You can either put your own needs on hold for awhile or think of something more interesting for Gemma to do in another room.

Early childhood education

Do children at preschool learn about their sexuality? They certainly do. Preschool is the first experience your child will have of an educational institution and it is often their first experience of learning about sexuality outside the family.

All early childhood centres in New Zealand are guided by a national curriculum that covers all areas of learning and development.[9] Programs at early childhood centres are based on principles of respect, caring and fairness.

Sexuality education is incorporated into these programs by encouraging children to:

1. Feel good about themselves and know their body is special.
2. Know the names of their body parts including the genitals. For example, the centre may have body jigsaws, anatomically correct dolls with a penis or vulva, and books on how the body works.
3. Know which parts of the body are private and should only be touched by those people caring for them.
4. Ask questions about their bodies, feelings, babies, and families and receive information about sexuality appropriate to their age.
5. Have equal opportunity to participate in activities. For example, ensuring girls and boys have equal access to equipment and games.

Teachers at preschool need clear policy guidelines in matters of privacy and nudity. However these policies should be sensitive to the needs of each child and the wishes of parents. For example, some children want to use the toilet with the door open, while others will insist on privacy. Flexibility from the teachers will allow these differences to be respected.

> *I was pleased to see the kindergarten teacher insist the children keep their clothes on when they played outside in the playground. I would have felt uncomfortable if they were allowed to run around in their underwear.*
>
> – Bernice, mother of Catrina, 3 years

> *When Nick was at Playcentre he would play with his friends in the water play area outside with no clothes on. I didn't mind them having no clothes on, but I worried that it was too cold and Nick would end up with another bout of asthma.*
>
> – Trudie, mother of Nick

Early childhood education is offered by a range of organisations, which differ in their educational philosophies, their approach to learning, and the way they involve parents. The following list includes the main choices available to parents in New Zealand:

- Playcentre. The centres are operated and staffed by parents. The Playcentre Federation organises comprehensive training for parents who wish to supervise children at their local Playcentre. Parental involvement is encouraged and children can attend from birth until they go to school.

- Kindergarten. Fully trained registered kindergarten teachers run programs for children from about 3½ years until they go to school. Parents are able to participate in kindergarten sessions by helping the teachers and the children.

- Te Kohunga Reo. The Kohunga is a total immersion Maori language and values program teaching children from birth until the children go to school. Professional development programs help teachers implement activities based on the curriculum.

- Montessori Preschool. Teachers trained in Dr Maria Montessori methods of teaching, design activities to stimulate the curiosity of children and allow them to learn by discovery. Ideally children attend the preschool for 3 years before they go to school.

- Rudolf Steiner Kindergarten. Learning is based on principles developed by Rudolf Steiner, an Austrian philosopher, scientist and educator. Children attend kindergarten until they are 7 years old. They learn in an environment where they play imaginatively and creatively and freely develop within their own world.

Try these with your pre-schooler

- Give your child plenty of opportunities to socialise with other boys and girls. They may get this experience at daycare, at preschool or at a neighbourhood playgroup. Start a playgroup yourself if they don't have one.

- Teach your pre-schooler about the public and private parts of the body, and public and private places. Explain that they can touch and look at the private parts of the body in a private place such as the bathroom or their bedroom, but not in a public place such as a supermarket.

- When playing with their dolls or soft toys show how they can express their feelings such as anger and frustration appropriately. If they are playing roughly, act out the consequences of getting hurt or in trouble.

- Reward 'friendly' behaviour such as sharing, making a new friend, or playing well with their friends.[9]

- Give your child their own photo album with photos of themselves from birth. Talk about how they have changed and the skills they have learnt. For example they can now put their toys away and dress themselves.

- Develop their sensuality by playing games with their eyes closed identifying objects by the way they feel, smell, sound and taste.

- Buy or borrow a book written for preschoolers about the differences between boys and girls, men and women, and how babies are made. Read the book with them just as you would other storybooks.

- You can help your child from an early age to become more independent. For example, let your preschooler decide which dress or sweater to wear, where to sit at the table, and so on. This will foster their decision-making skills and encourage independence.

8

Primary school children

Lisa has now been at school a year. I am amazed at how quickly she is learning to read and write her own stories. She still needs help to tie her own shoelaces but is getting more independent in other ways. She has joined a gymnastics class after school. Like the other young gymnasts she vaults, flips and tumbles, not without her fair share of bumps and bruises.

-Don, Lisa's father

By the time your child starts school they will have mastered many basic physical skills. Like Lisa they will go on to develop and refine movements required for complex activities such as tying shoe laces, writing, swimming, gymnastics or playing football. In this 5 to 9 year age range your child will learn complicated concepts, learn to reason and develop problem-solving skills. They understand the difference between male and female. Their social development moves ahead rapidly.

Social development

At school your child will mix with a wide range of children and learn to work and play with others, some of who will become friends and some they won't like. They learn about themselves. They begin to develop an awareness of what others think of them and how their own behaviour can effect others. They become aware that other people may not think the same way as they do, that they may have different ideas and different opinions. They learn to consider the needs of others. They form closer friendships, play after school with their friends and may stay overnight with them.

Your child will focus more on same sex friendships. Boys now prefer to play with boys and girls with girls. Sex play is common at this age within these same-sex groups. Sometimes they will look at and touch each other's genitals. This is normal behaviour and does not influence your child's future sexual orientation. In these situations your child is simply exploring and developing an awareness of their sexuality which will help give them knowledge and confidence about their bodies. Without that information they may grow up feeling that their bodies are embarrassing, dirty, and different from everyone else's.

Sex play between boys and girls may also begin to include kissing games, teasing and pretend games about marriage. At age 8 or 9 it is common for children to start talking about girlfriends and boyfriends. It is unusual for these first relationships to be serious. There is much talk about who is 'going out' with who, even though they rarely talk to each other, let alone go out together.

Learning about gender

Why do boys have a penis? Why do girls have a vagina?

By the age of six or seven your child knows that they are either a girl or a boy and that this will not change. They are now very aware of the differences between the sexes and ask questions about them.[10] If your child doesn't have the opportunity to learn about the differences between male and female at this age they may become obsessively curious at a later time. So you have work to do. By the time they go to school they need to know what the acceptable words are for the sexual parts of the body, and what the acceptable sexual words are within the family. They also need to know the language others could use. Your child is at risk of being teased by others if they use words they don't understand and make silly mistakes.

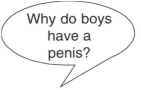

Tracey, 5 years, was being teased at school by the boys chanting, "Tracey's got a vagina, Tracey's got a vagina." She indignantly told them that she didn't have a vagina. Later in front of the class she told her male teacher that the boys kept saying she had a vagina even when she told them she hadn't. Although the teacher handled the situation very well Tracey was embarrassed that she hadn't known what the boys had been talking about.

Showing affection and sharing intimacy

Primary school children continue to need the hugs and cuddles they did before they went to school. Sometimes they seem to regress to behaving like preschoolers, curling up in your lap and sucking their thumb or climbing into bed with you to share your intimacy and warmth.

When we visit Bruce's parents, Bruce insists that the children give Nanna and Pop a kiss when we arrive. They try to avoid it and complain about it later. I don't think they should have to do it if they don't want to.

-Gail, mother of two

Children have a right not to let other people hug or touch them if it makes them feel uncomfortable. Bruce had an expectation that his children would kiss their grandparents on family visits. Expecting children to show this affection when they feel uneasy about it is unfair. It would be hypocritical to teach them their body is special and they are in control of it if you also expect them to show affection when they feel uncomfortable about it.

As they get older they will find other ways to experience closeness such as cuddling up beside you on the couch when watching television or asking you to give them a back massage. If they don't ask, try to create opportunities for this to happen. However you need to respect the limits they put on this intimacy.

Rules and setting boundaries

Children feel confident when they know that what they say and believe is important to you. Work out rules together and help them to follow them. Arguments will be reduced if your child knows that they must always sit in the back seat of the car, or that the rule is that they can only have two cookies after school. Work out a roster together and allocate easy-to-achieve jobs, for example: feeding the cat, setting the table, taking out the rubbish.

> *The kids used to barge straight into my bedroom and I was sick of it. So we made a rule that they had to knock. They agreed as long as we did the same for them. That's fair really.*
> -Paul, father of three[11]

Their sense of fairness is developing. They will compare the way you treat them with how others are treated to decide if you are being fair with them.

> *It's not fair that I have to go to bed at 8 o'clock, Ryan is allowed to stay up 'til 9.*
> -Tuiri, 6-year-old

You can explain that different families have different family rules. School children also learn that games are governed by rules.

A 6 year old in a group of girls playing weddings says, "You can't marry Gina 'cos you're a girl and you're not allowed and you'll get into trouble if you do that".

Children will develop their own set of rules for an activity if there are none. At this age children believe authority is always right and if you don't follow the rules or misbehave you get punished.[12] They learn about acceptable ways to behave and begin to make moral judgements about others. They may be on the receiving end of teasing or bullying at school, or start to tease and bully other children.

This is the time to talk about and to set clear boundaries. Primary school children can understand that boundaries are sets of rules about personal space. Start by teaching your child that their body is special. They can control who they let touch them or be close to them, and they have a right to be treated with respect.

Since she started school Lisa is embarrassed if I see her getting changed. It's the opposite to a year or so ago when she used to run around the house with nothing on.

-Don, Lisa's father

By the age of six or seven your child may be embarrassed about nudity. There could be a growing modesty in front of you as well as others. When your child starts school they will usually know that sex games, looking at each other's bodies and masturbation are things people do in private.

Among themselves children find bathroom and toilet jokes very amusing. How you respond to this will depend on your own values and where you set the limits. For example, in some families when parents overhear these jokes they pretend they didn't. If they offend you or become a problem you can say they can have their private jokes but you don't want to hear them.

Touching the genitals

Fay shared this story about her son at a parent evening:

> *John had developed a habit of holding onto his penis when he was anxious as a young child and continued to do it occasionally during his junior school years. He seemed unaware of the behaviour. Jane found it embarrassing and hoped he would stop but didn't say anything to him about it.*
>
> *When John was nine years old he had written a prize-winning speech and was asked to repeat the speech at the end of year prize giving. Standing up in front of the assembly of children and parents he gave his speech, with one hand firmly holding his penis. Jane felt so embarrassed for him as she heard the whispering and sniggering from his schoolmates. Now she wishes she had helped him by bringing it to his attention when it first occurred.*

If your child is often touching or holding their genitals at age 6 or 7 it is probably because something is worrying them. Try to work out what the problem is. Telling your child who is masturbating for comfort not to do so is likely to make them more anxious. Try saying, "I can see you are feeling worried about something, come and I'll give you hug."

When a 4-year-old is under stress it is common for them to hold their genitals and to have the urge to relieve themselves. It may have become a habit by the time they start school. You can discourage this by quietly raising their awareness when it occurs so that the behaviour doesn't persist.

Bedwetting

All children wet their beds occasionally. Bedwetting is defined as a problem when it occurs more than one night a month. It is very common, occurring in 10% of 6-year-olds and 3% of 12-year-olds.[13]

A small bladder capacity, deep sleeping or a number of medical reasons may cause bedwetting. It is more commonly a problem for boys and often runs in families. It can be very helpful for a child to know that it was also a problem for one of their parents. They will know their parents understand how they are feeling.

Staying overnight with a friend or going on a school camp can cause extra anxiety for these children. The problem may cause considerable tension within families and embarrassment for the child. Even the most understanding parents can become frustrated and angry with repeated accidents and need extra support. If the problem persists until the child is 7 years old, behavior management techniques or medication can be helpful. In this case the first step is to talk to a health professional.

Intercourse, pregnancy and birth

How does a baby come out Mum? How does the baby get in?

Do these questions throw you? Don't let them. They are asked out of curiosity. Your child is interested in the facts of pregnancy and birth, they are not asking about sexual feelings. Most 6 and 7-year-olds imagine babies are somehow manufactured by adults, like supermarket items. However they do seem to realise that both sexes are required.

My friend says a man puts his penis in a lady's vagina......but it's not true really.

-Darryn, 7 years[14]

Darryn is not sure who or what to believe. Children hear about sexual intercourse and talk about it among themselves. They often use sex words they have heard from their friends but they may not know what the words mean. This is the beginning of sex talk and joking about sex with peers. They are old enough to understand sexual intercourse if you explain it to them when the opportunity arises.

If your child asks the question, "How are babies made?" a simple answer is to explain in your own words that when a man and a woman are loving each other in a special way the man puts his penis in the woman's vagina. Some fluid comes out of the penis with sperm in it. The sperm look for an egg cell inside the woman. If they meet a new baby starts to grow.

They may go on to ask questions about how they will be boys or girls, ask when they are getting a baby sister and are often fascinated by anything unusual, such as Siamese twins. Don't be surprised if children think sexual activity sounds either ridiculous or disgusting. When a boy saw a couple kissing passionately on a park bench he asked what they were doing. He was told they were kissing and he said, "Yuk, I'm never going to do that!" He has plenty of time to change his mind.

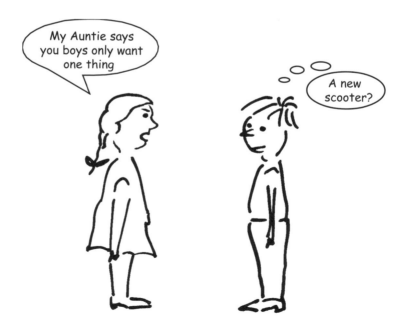

Learning about sex, love and relationships

*Simon (6 years) asked his mother what a wet dream was.
His mother asked him what he had heard about wet dreams
and he said, "A wet dream is when something spooky and
scary sneaks in to your bed on a dark night".* [15]

Where could Simon have picked up this notion? He has been listening
to others and has 'put two and two together' and this is his spooky
conclusion. Children see sexual behaviour in one way or another
through television, videos and magazines. They read, see and hear
about what it means to be a man or a woman, and how men and
women behave. They often end up with misunderstandings.
Sometimes they see pictures of sexual violence and other sexual
activity that they are not old enough to understand. Your child is
influenced by these images. Keep in touch with what they are
watching on TV and talk about issues as they arise. You will be
more likely to clarify something that your child may have found
confusing or disturbing at the time it occurs rather than trying to
piece it together later.

From about age 6 children begin to develop a concept of love and
identify the people who love them. They may worry that if they are
naughty they may lose your love. You can help by being clear that
when your child does something you don't like, it is the behaviour
you don't like, not them.

*Matt's 7 year old son Peter kept asking for reassurance that
Matt would always love him and always love Carolyn, Peter's
mother. After this happened a few times Matt asked Peter if
he was worried that they would stop loving him. Peter then
told him about a classmate whose parents had recently
separated and Peter was worried that it might happen to his
family.*

If children see their parents or other adults constantly putting each other down or making fun of people of the opposite sex, they learn that one sex is better than the other. They may in turn feel unhappy about being a boy or a girl. Or they may feel they are better than the opposite sex. Sometimes they become afraid or wary of people of the other sex.

Georgina wanted to be a boy from the age of 3 or 4. She even went through a stage of only answering if called George. She liked to play with boys and refused to wear dresses or play with girls. Soon after starting school she began to accept that she was a girl and started to develop closer friendships with the other girls.

You want your child to have a healthy attitude toward sex and the fact that they are a boy or girl. The way you behave or react in any talk about sex and men and women will affect how they think and feel. At this age you can take opportunities to tell your child what your values and attitudes are about sexuality and relationships, without turning it into a lecture. Do this in a low-key friendly way rather than being earnest or moralistic. Having open communication about sexuality issues will make it easier for your child to ask questions and make it more likely that they will talk to you when they are teenagers.

Discovered during sex

You are in the throes of a vigorous session of lovemaking and in walks your child. Sound familiar? It happens to many of us. Don't worry, it would be unusual for them to see anything that could be disturbing for them. School children are old enough to understand that you need to have some time privately, and to be asked to go and find something else to do. If you do intend to explore exotic techniques and sexual fantasies it would be a good idea to lock the bedroom door.

Encouraging independence

You can help your child feel that they have control over their lives by helping them make decisions and then supporting those decisions. When they suffer the consequences of what later appears to have been a wrong decision remember that the decision was the right one for them when they made it. They need your support rather than being told they made the wrong decision.

> *When Kean (7 years) was invited to play at Jimmy's house for the day he couldn't make up his mind if he wanted to go. Kean's father, Sam, helped him to think about the pros and cons of the decision. The positives included: having a friend to play with all day; not getting bored at home; getting to swim at Jimmy's pool; getting to know Jimmy better. The negatives included: not being able to come home early if he wanted to (he had to wait until Sam finished work); having to put up with Jimmy's annoying little sister; having to eat their kind of food at lunch time; and risking arguing with Jimmy and not being able to work it out. Kean weighed up the pros and cons and decided to go.*
>
> *He found the day very long and was pleased when Sam came to collect him. "I shouldn't have gone," he said miserably to his father. Sam reminded him that he had thought about it carefully and he had decided that the best thing would be to go. Sam explained that even when you think carefully before making decisions, sometimes the decision doesn't seem to have been the right one. However Kean had known the consequence would be that he would have to wait until after work to be collected.*

Kean had done well to manage as well as he did. He had learned some valuable lessons for himself that would help him make decisions in the future.

Puberty approaches

Puberty is not far away. In some children the first changes can start as early as age 7 or 8. Look out for the early changes leading up to puberty. The next chapter deals with puberty in detail, but here is a story of an early developer:

> *Carol, 8 years old, complained that she didn't want to go swimming at school because she had to get changed into her swimsuit in front of the other girls. Her father Sam stated strongly that she shouldn't be ashamed of her body and that she was being ridiculous. He didn't realise that she had started to develop breasts and pubic hair, and was feeling uncomfortable because her friends hadn't.*

For Sam nudity among people of the same sex is natural and he thought Carol shouldn't be ashamed of her body. He didn't know Carol had already started to develop breasts. It would have been more helpful if Sam had listened to Carol and found out why she was embarrassed. Girls can be very self-consciousness at this time, and need reassurance that they are developing normally. If he had known he could have reassured her that other girls would be starting to develop soon, and she could be proud that she was one of the first.

Try these with your 5-9 year old

- Draw patterns or write words with your finger on your child's back and ask them to guess what they are.
- Gently rub your child's back or the back of their neck when they are upset, anxious or feeling unwell.
- Read books together about differences between girls and boys.
- Teach them the proper names for the sexual parts of the body if you haven't already – by the time they start school.
- Support and encourage physical and sporting interests.
- Create opportunities for intimacy with you – sitting on a couch reading a book, playing games, even computer games, if you sit side by side so you have contact.
- Encourage your child to make or draw something to give as a present or a get well gift.
- Let your child know that we all have problems and that talking about them helps us to work out what to do. For example, your 8-year-old son needs to move out of his room while his grandparents come to stay. Help him work out what he will need for school the next day so that he doesn't need to disturb them early in the morning.
- Dad - try not to set standards too high or your son will never feel he is good enough in your eyes. Your son has lots to learn, physically and intellectually, so don't expect him to be as good as you are or were at his age. For example, if he is too frightened to go on the waterslide and bursts into tears he needs your support. If you tell him not to be silly, or not to act like a baby, he will feel put down. If you tell him that you were scared when you first went on the slide and that you will be right behind him he will feel he has your support.

9

Puberty – physical and emotional changes

Suddenly our little boy with pins for legs just shot up. He ate like a horse, couldn't walk down the hall without banging into the walls, his voice was all croaky, and he had that adolescent boy smell. Even his face seemed to change shape - his nose looked out of proportion to the rest of his face. It took a few years before he regained control of his body.

-Maria, mother of a teenage son

What was puberty like for you? Intense sexual feelings, excitement and fun, greasy hair and zits, uncertainty and embarrassment. All of these and more. It'll be like that for your child too. You, like Maria, may be surprised by the sudden growth spurt that often occurs at puberty. Puberty may start as early as 8 years old and continue well into the teenage years.

What's happening? Puberty is the time when young people start to change from being a child to an adult. It usually starts two to three years earlier for girls than boys. The outward signs of sexual maturity appear first, breast buds and pubic hair. Boys testes enlarge and begin producing sperm. Girls begin menstruating about a year after breast development first appears. Hormones are sent from the pituitary gland in the brain to the testicles in boys and ovaries in girls. These hormones are chemical messages that cause the testicles and ovaries to release other hormones. The hormones work together to trigger the changes associated with puberty.[16]

What are the physical changes?

Your child gets taller, heavier and stronger. They can have heaps of energy one day and be exhausted the next. All this growing needs fuel. Parents of children going through puberty will recognise the common complaint of "There's never any food in the house". They crave for lots of carbohydrates and food that can be prepared instantly to satisfy this amazing hunger. This from a 12 year old:

I get so hungry I'll eat anything, even stuff I don't even like.

Zits? The hormones cause an increase in sweating and oiliness of the skin. This can be a problem and cause zits or pimples on the face and other parts of the body. It can be uncomfortable and look unsightly. Young people can be very self-conscious with even the smallest problem. Washing with hot water is better than squeezing and prodding pimples, which can introduce infection. Drinking plenty of water and eating lots of fruit and vegetables will help, but if there is a major problem talk to a nurse or doctor about it. There are many treatments available including using mild cleansing agents, applying antibiotic creams, or taking a course of oral antibiotics.

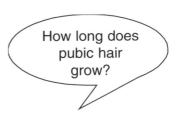

How long does pubic hair grow?

They become hairy. Hair grows around the genitals, under the arms and on the legs and arms. There is an increase in the size of the genitals. They are more likely to masturbate, or rub their genitals for pleasure. They are more modest, want more privacy and need time to themselves.

Some young people feel unattractive and worry that they can't make friends easily. They may start blaming all the bits of their body that don't look right, thinking that if they change their appearance everyone will like them.

> *No one likes me. I am fat and have huge ugly stretch marks on my breasts and hips and stomach. My body is so ugly that I could never ever show anyone. I will never be able to get married. I feel like a bloated cow. Someone called me that once. Is there anything I can do? Please help me.*
> - Sandra, 12 years, in a letter to a sexuality educator

This 12-year-old is feeling depressed about what has happened to her body. The number of children who are obese is increasing. The most common cause of obesity is diet related rather than due to a medical condition. Promoting a good diet and encouraging regular exercise will help prevent excessive weight gain. If your child is not interested in organised sport, suggest walking to school or swimming. At this age obese children are often teased by classmates and they may develop poor self esteem. They need your ongoing support to help them cope with their condition. The best thing you can do for an overweight child is to get professional advice early. Evidence shows that if intervention is provided early in the course of obesity, weight control is likely to be more successful.[17]

The physical changes at this age take a bit of getting used to. Their body image takes time to adjust. You too will have some adjusting to do, as your child will probably soon be looking down on you.

Emotional changes

Your child may have stormy waves of emotion or sail calmly through puberty. However most young people experience sudden mood swings and intense emotions - love, hate, jealousy, joy, anger, sadness.

They can feel passionately about issues that they weren't aware of a few years before.

Throughout puberty young people may think that everyone is looking at them as if they are 'on stage' or in a fishbowl. Life revolves around them. They are the centre of the universe. They may believe that nothing bad will ever happen to them. Their parents seem to worry endlessly about possible problems and situations that to them don't exist. They are excited by the possibilities life now offers and don't want to miss out.

An increase in sexual feelings and fantasies may cause them to blush in almost any situation. Most young people at this age are aware of sexual feelings and attractions for others, for the same sex and the opposite sex. If they feel attracted to the same sex it doesn't mean they will necessarily be gay or lesbian. They need reassurance that these feelings are normal during adolescence.

Encourage them to talk about what they are feeling - even if it may be that they just feel like being alone and not talking at that moment. Be patient with their moodiness and swings of emotion.

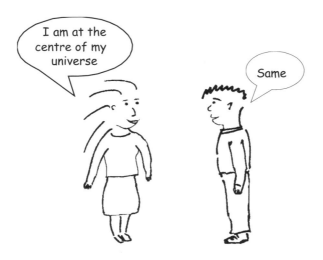

What's happening socially?

Spending more time with their friends than their family is common. They start to question family values and have definite ideas of their own. As their independence increases they become increasingly preoccupied with what other people of the same age think of them. They may feel pressure from their friends to do and look like they do.[18] When they are with their friends they may change their minds and their plans every few minutes.

There may be conflicting pressures from two sides. Their friends may be saying one thing, and Mum and Dad the opposite. For example, you may encourage your son to do the best he can at school. However he wants to be like his other classmates and is reluctant to appear too smart.

In a similar way, you expect your child to be honest and always tell the truth, but there may be pressure from their friends not to be a goodie-goodie. This can cause conflict and confusion. On the one hand they still want to please you but on the other they don't want to lose face with their friends. You need to be aware of this dilemma and show that you understand what is happening. Explaining why you believe what you do will help. Parents are still the main source of values, so continue letting your child know where you stand on issues.

How can you help?

Changes during puberty can leave young people feeling uneasy and confused. Give them lots of reassurance that these changes are normal. Your child is growing up but they are not necessarily growing away from you.

Young people need help to see themselves as people with their own ideas, feelings and personality. Tell them people don't judge them only on their appearance. Point out your child's good qualities and show them that you value what they do and say. It is also important for young people to be with friends who accept them for who they are.

Making sure your child has interests outside school and that they have plenty of opportunities to mix with people of their own age will help them find friends who are supportive and compatible. Encourage them to develop their interests in some way to keep physically fit. People who exercise regularly generally feel better about themselves. Exercising is also a way for them to keep in touch with their changing shape and to gain control over their body. Look for a sport or activity that will suit their physique and temperament.

> *11 year old Tania was invited to her best friend Sandra's house for Sandra's birthday. All her friends were going to sleep over. For Tania it was a hard decision to make, as she was sure her period was due to start that night. It would only be her third period, and she felt unsure she could manage. After pondering the question all day, she finally asked her mother to collect her from the party at 9.30pm.*
>
> *Next day her period had not started, and her friends talked excitedly about the great time they had at the party. She complained moodily to her Mum that she had made the wrong decision and missed out on the fun.*

Like Tania, your daughter may have trouble making decisions when learning to manage her periods. You can help by working through the pros and cons of the various options with her.

What are the changes girls will experience?

At the time girls start to grow pubic hair their breasts are usually starting to develop. The nipple area swells first and later the whole breast develops. Periods usually begin a year after this. Often one breast develops faster than the other. Girls need to know that this is normal.

Girls notice their vulva gets bigger and softer. They often have a vaginal discharge - an increase in the mucus produced in the vagina. They may be wondering if other girls have the same 'white stuff' on their pants or if they have as much mucus as they do. When feeling aroused the vagina gets wetter too. At this age girls may have an orgasm if they masturbate. Explain to your daughter she can expect to have a discharge and she may find her pants feel quite wet. Give her small pads or pantishields to use if necessary.

Your daughter will start to change shape, with more rounded hips and a more defined waist. Girls worry that they may get fat or may already be too fat. They also worry if people say they are skinny. Teaching girls about a balanced diet, healthy foods and regular exercise is important. Many young girls go on diets to lose weight, which inevitably cause them to gain weight when they stop. You may worry that she is preoccupied with how she looks. Girls can be very critical of their bodies and not like the size they are. They can become very focussed on specific details. Here is a typical conversation between two friends:

Sheila, 11 years: *"My thighs are so fat."*

Helen, 11 years: *"Same. Look at my ankles. I don't even have ankles. See how your legs go in at the ankles. Why don't mine do that?"*

Sheila: *"I've got cellulite. Look at my cellulite. How do I get rid of it? It's so gross."*

You can help your daughter realise that her body knows what shape and size it needs to be. Explain that she can't change her basic body shape.

Some girls worry that everyone else seems to want to have a boyfriend and they aren't interested. They may think boys are silly or immature. Girls are curious about the changes boys go through and have many questions about their development such as how long do penises grow, how long erections last, and what causes boys to have wet dreams. Make opportunities to talk about the changes boys will experience as well as the changes at puberty for girls.

Menstruation

I wanted my daughter to feel really special when her period started, and to feel that it is an important milestone to becoming a woman. But I couldn't help also feeling sad it would be the end of her childhood and that precious childhood innocence.

-Belinda, mother of Stacey, 12 years

My mother tells me it will be a special, amazing time when my period starts but it's also kind of scary waiting for it to happen. It's embarrassing. Why do girls have to have them anyway?

-Stacey

Belinda told Stacey that having periods is an important milestone in becoming a woman, and it is. However, your daughter has many milestones to go and the message that she is now a woman is misleading. She may still be a child in the other areas of her development.

Girls start their periods when they weigh about 41 kilos (90 pounds) and are about 149cms (4 foot 10) tall. It is usually between 9 and 14 years. Studies show that height is the most reliable predictor of when a girl can expect to have her first period.[19] Each period lasts for 2 to 7 days. Her periods may be irregular at first but usually settle down to a pattern after a few months. If your daughter hasn't started her period by the time she is 16 it would be a good idea to talk to a nurse or doctor about it.

Your daughter may wonder what her period will be like and worry that it may start with a flood in the middle of the day. You can tell her that doesn't usually happen. She will usually notice a small amount of blood and mucus when she gets up in the morning. However she could take some spare underwear and a pad in her school bag or overnight bag if she is staying away from home.

Girls usually experience some period pain and sometimes it can be severe. It may be low back pain, pelvic pain and may radiate down the legs. Some girls have an upset stomach, feel nauseous or even vomit on the first day of their period. These symptoms are usually caused by the release of a hormone called prostaglandins. Medication is available to reduce the amount of prostaglandins released and is therefore more effective if taken 12 - 24 hours before the period starts.

Buy a supply of pads for your daughter so that she is prepared. She may wish to try using tampons after managing her first periods using pads. At night it is safer to continue to use pads, as tampons need to be changed every 3-4 hours. A common misconception is that women cannot use tampons until after they have experienced sexual intercourse. They are able to use tampons even when their hymen is intact. The hymen is a piece of skin inside and partially closing the vagina. At puberty the hymen will often already be stretched open through normal physical activity.

> *My mother told me nothing about periods, so when it happened I freaked out. I don't want that to happen to my daughter but I don't know how to say it. It's a big culture issue for us.*
>
> -Mele, Samoan mother

> *I was lucky 'cos my nanny told me about my mate (period) and mate rags (sanitary pads) so when it came time to talk*

*to my girls it was okay for me. But most of my friends didn't
know about it 'til it happened. You only talked about those
things down there with your husband.*

-Moana, Maori mother of three girls

Most women know of other women who weren't prepared for
their first period. The unexpected bleeding can shock girls. Some
may think they have cancer or are dying because of the pain and
bleeding. Some girls feel they are being punished.

If you find it difficult to talk to your daughter try talking to other
mothers about it first. Young girls want to hear about periods from
their mothers, and their early personal experiences of them.
Alternatively tell your daughter you are finding it hard to talk about
this because it is such a sensitive and important issue. She will
appreciate your honesty and you will find it much easier once you
get started. If you talk to your daughter and she seems uninterested
be sure to come back later and show her you are comfortable
answering questions.

What are the changes boys will experience?

If you use your penis a lot will it stop functioning?

-Tim, 10 years, during a puberty health program at school

Boys' shoulders and chests become broader and their muscles get
bigger. Their penis and testicles will also enlarge. By this age your
son should be able to retract his foreskin. He will probably compare
the size of his penis with others to see if he is normal. He will have
seen an adult penis, for example his father's penis, and may wonder
if his will ever get that big. He will have more erections, sometimes
for no apparent reason. He may wonder if other boys can control
their erections, and be embarrassed if he thinks others may notice he
has an erection.

Sperm will start to be produced in his testicles at about the time that he starts to grow pubic hair. This will usually be between 11 and 16 years. He can now ejaculate and/or reach orgasm when masturbating. Your son may have wet dreams, that is, ejaculate in his sleep. He may or may not remember it happening.

> *I woke in the morning to find my pyjamas wet and sticky. I thought there was something wrong, that I was sick. I wanted to tell Mum but I couldn't. At school I sort of hinted to the other boys about it and found out about it that way.*
> -Steve, now 15, recalling his first wet dream at age 11

Hair starts to grow on your son's face and sometimes his chest. Shaving is a new experience. Initially there will be just a few hairs on his upper lip and chin that need removing once a week. He will need his own shaver and shaving cream. Fathers can show their son the finer points of shaving, and this is an opportunity to open a conversation about the other changes ahead.

Boys voices will get deeper. Sometimes this can be difficult for them. Their voice may go up and down or sound croaky all in one sentence. Occasionally they may start to speak and not be able to get any sound out at all. Some boys may have a temporary swelling of the breasts as their hormones sort themselves out. This can cause anxiety and they need reassurance that it is normal and they are not really growing breasts.

Boys are curious about girls physical development. Their own development usually starts later than girls. They notice that girls of the same age are much more developed sexually than they are and may be slightly intimidated by this. Girl's periods, breast development and moody behaviour all seem to have occurred suddenly and this can be mysterious to boys. Explaining these changes to your son will remove some of this mystery.

They become interested in any material they can find which may tell them about sex, ranging from soft porn magazines and TV, to explicit material available on pay TV, video and the Internet. Technology is available to block access to web sites and TV channels, however if you are too controlling young people aren't learning to make their own decisions. It can also make them more determined to access it. However we try to limit access to pornography, young people can be exposed outside the home through their friends, teenagers and others. Even if you don't think this is a possibility for your child, the open communication you have developed will enable them to talk to you if they are exposed to pornography and are disturbed by what they have seen.

Try these with your 9 – 12-year-old

- Hang out together. Spend time sharing your interests and your feelings with your child. Really listen and acknowledge their ideas and feelings. Show them respect. Also spend time together doing the things they want you to, even when it is something you are not usually interested in.
- Continue to show affection - particularly with your sons. Everyone needs to be hugged. However if your child goes through a stage of rejecting your touch, respect the boundaries they are setting.
- Look out for books, magazines, pamphlets and articles you think may be of interest and leave them in places you know they will see them. If you make a point of giving them something to read don't demand anything in return. You could bring up the subject later by saying that you found it interesting and give your reasons but you may be disappointed if you expect feedback.
- Buy your daughter a supply of pads and tampons for her to experiment with. Suggest ways to cope with the unexpected, for example if she finds her period starts at school or at a friend's house. Also explain how to dispose of the pad after she has used it to avoid the embarrassment of a blocked toilet.
- Suggest your daughter use a mirror to get to know the sexual parts of her body. Explain that the sexual areas such as the clitoris and the vagina are external while the reproductive areas such as the uterus and the ovaries are protected well inside the body.
- Give lots of reassurance and praise and show you appreciate your child's good qualities.

10

Preparing your child for puberty

I was only 9 when my period started. I freaked out. I didn't know what was happening to me. I couldn't ask my mother. We never talked of such things.

-Senata, Fijian girl in New Zealand

Talking to your child before puberty about the upcoming physical and emotional changes is very important. Use the techniques and tips in the *Ask me anything* section to help. It is more difficult if you have been taught that talking about sexual issues is taboo in your culture. You face a dilemma deciding whether or not you break this taboo. We think you should consider your child's interests first. By talking you can reduce the risk of them feeling alone and anxious like Senata with her first period.

Reassure your child that puberty can begin as early as 8 or as late as 15 or older. This will offset any anxiety if they don't start at the same age as their friends and classmates.

Donna's 16-year-old daughter Lisa has always been small for her age. Lisa has a huge appetite but never seems to put on weight. At the age her friends had started puberty her mother talked to her about how lucky she was that her period wouldn't start until she was much older than her friends. Lisa says she is pleased that she is free of those worries but Donna can't help but wonder how she really feels about being different from her girlfriends.

It can also be difficult for those girls who develop earlier than their peers.

Theresa started her period when she was 10 years old, about one year before her friends. She didn't admit to the others that she had started menstruating until some of them had started too.

Children need lots of reassurance that their development is normal. Here is a typical example:

Nathan (12 years) was concerned that he was developing breasts. His father Elias had noticed this, and had called a medical friend, who assured him that one in ten boys get some breast development at puberty, which settles down later. Elias was able to reassure Nathan that this was a normal occurrence.

Don't ignore concerns that appear trivial, and treat all concerns with confidentiality.

Kelly (11 years) told her mother Catherine she was worried that one of her breasts was getting bigger than the other. Catherine brought up the subject with some of her women friends at work during morning coffee, and she was relieved to hear that a number of them had the same experience during puberty. When Catherine told Kelly this later, she was surprised that Kelly was upset that she had discussed her concern with others.

Young people can feel that their trust has been betrayed when their parents talk about them to their friends. It is good to share things with friends but your child needs to realise that just as they share things with each other, parents need to too. You could agree not to share without your child's permission. It is important for you to get the support you need.

Women's magazines and magazines for teenagers have information about health, sexuality and development. Girls often have access to these magazines. Girls also talk amongst themselves about these issues but boys can often feel very isolated. The most anxiety comes from not knowing how others are coping with these changes. Everyone else can look like they've got it all under control.

Fathers and sons

Children need to have a trusted adult they can talk to. Parents most often fill this role exclusively until puberty. However following puberty it is difficult for a father to fill this role with his son. This is because boys at this age see themselves in competition with their fathers. Fathers are their primary role model for what it is to be a man. Boys struggle to be as good as their fathers, who are inevitably

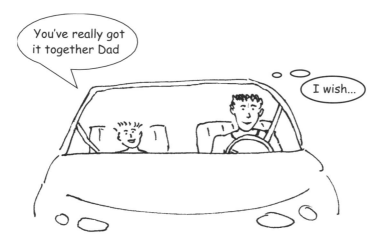

stronger, wiser, more skilled and have 'got it together' in a way boys can only dream about. This makes it very difficult for boys to turn to their fathers with their personal problems.[20]

Make sure your son knows other men care for him - an uncle, coach, a male teacher, or a family friend. And whether you are his father or mother, let your son know you are open to talking about sexual matters and provide him with written information. The *Further Reading* section at the end of this book lists useful resources.

Attitudes to sex

Here is an interesting fact: young people are curious about sex. Of course you knew that. Their interest is normal and healthy. They have many questions and they may or may not ask you for answers. Here are

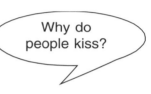

Why do people kiss?

some examples of questions young people of this age placed in an anonymous question box at school during a health course. They will give you an idea of the questions that your child may have:

How do people have sex?

When is the right time to have sex?

Why do people kiss?

Does it hurt when a boy puts his dick up a girl's fanny?

Is sex dirty?

How would you know what hole to put it in?

Can you get stuck in the vagina?

What is a blowjob?

Is it okay to have sex at a young age?

Why is sex such a big deal for adults? They won't talk about it or go bananas if we talk about it.

What will you say if your son or daughter asks when you first had sex, how often you have sex or how many people you have had sex with? When your child asks personal questions think about how much you want to disclose. They don't need to know your personal details but they still want answers. Try to answer them in a general way. For example you could tell them that some people have sex every day at one stage in their lives and may have sex once a month at other times in their lives. The next section, *Ask me anything,* gives ideas on how to answer these questions.

Puberty and disability

Puberty is a time when young people are learning to be independent from their parents and are taking more responsibility for themselves. This is difficult for children with disabilities and for their parents. Many people, including parents, find it hard to acknowledge that people with disabilities have or experience sexuality. As the parent of a child with a disability, you may be confronted for the first time with the realisation that they are growing up. You don't want to see your child taken advantage of by others and you want to keep them safe. The more severe the disability, the stronger the protective feelings are likely to be.

Nearly all young people going through puberty perceive their parents to be over-protective and restrictive. If they have a disability they may feel this more strongly and feel that their parents continue to treat them like children. Puberty is a time when young people are self conscious and very aware of their appearance. They want to appear the same as their friends. Young people who depend on mobility aids or other people for their basic needs are at a disadvantage because they look different.

Ensuring your child looks good and is offered the same opportunities as others their age will help them develop positive feelings about growing up. Learning to tie shoe laces with one hand or teaching a child who is regularly catheterised that their genitals are private can present a huge challenge for parents. Your child will appreciate your efforts to help them fit in with their friends. For example, it is possible to find trendy clothes that are also comfortable when sitting in a wheelchair or to arrange for friends to stay overnight with them.

Menstruation and disability

Menstruation can present specific challenges to parents of girls with a disability.

- *Physical disability*. There may be practical difficulties managing sanitary pads and tampons, particularly if there is already a need to wear pads for incontinence. Wherever possible girls need to be independent when managing their periods.
- *Intellectual disability*. Girls need to be prepared well before their periods start. The sight of blood may be frightening, as blood is usually associated with being hurt. They need to practice wearing pads and have a clear checklist of steps to go through for changing them.[21] Oral or injectable contraception may be a useful way to control or stop menstruation as they get older.

Early sexual development

You will have seen reports in the media that children are reaching sexual maturity earlier than previous generations. The average age of menstruation has fallen over the past 100 years from 17 to about 13 years. Some girls begin breast development very early, as early as 7 years old. A study by Bristol University's Institute of Child Health found one in six British girls reach puberty by eight years of age, and half of all girls in Britain enter puberty by the age of 10.[22] Another finding was that one in 14 eight-year-old boys had pubic hair, compared with one in 150 boys of their fathers generation.

Paediatricians are concerned at the trend toward earlier puberty and researchers have many theories about it. Some suggest hormones in meat may be responsible. Others blame industrial or agricultural chemicals such as PCBs, DDT or certain types of plastics, which can have hormone-like effects. Children are more likely to be overweight and taller than 50 years ago. Other reasons suggested are the sexualized messages on TV, in music, movies and advertising. Whatever the cause, if you notice your child developing sexually at 7 years or younger you should talk to a health professional.

Recognising possible problems

Apart from early sexual development or other medical conditions, there are other times when your child could need professional help. How would you know if they have emotional or social difficulties? You would probably notice a worrying change in their behaviour. You are the best person to recognise a change because you know your child better than anyone.

Use the following list of disturbing behaviours as a guide when making a decision about seeking help. Any of these behaviours may typically describe your child some of the time and doesn't necessarily mean they have a problem. For example, if your child has sleeping problems for a week, that is not unusual. If the problem persists for a few weeks or more, you need to seek advice.

You may notice that:

- They have become very quiet, submissive, tearful or never stand up for themselves
- They have become aggressive and rude, not only to you and other adults but also to their friends. They don't care how their behaviour is affecting others
- They have become vague, distracted or have difficulty concentrating
- They want to sleep all the time or have difficulty sleeping
- They lose their appetite, refuse to eat, eat constantly or become obsessed with their weight

- They lose interest in their appearance, express feelings of self doubt, feel inferior or appear depressed
- They become obsessed with a belief that could be harmful to others. For example, that they have a right to harass gay men because they believe homosexuality is obscene.

During puberty many children are moody or have mood swings. But if one mood persists it may be a problem. Share your concerns with your child. This will give them an opportunity to talk. You may want to talk about it with other parents to put the behaviour in perspective. If you continue to be concerned do not hesitate to talk to a counsellor, nurse or doctor.

Sexual experimentation

Because children are reaching sexual maturity earlier than ever before, boys and girls are physiologically capable of sexual activity before they are ready emotionally. Give your child a clear message that sexual intercourse is an adults-only activity. They are far too young to experience sex.

Between the ages of 10 and 12 some children do experiment with sexual intercourse and oral sex. It tends to be a purely physical activity and often occurs in groups. The boys "see if it will fit". They take turns with the others watching. Sometimes it is a result of a dare, part of a game or they are bullied into it. They risk pregnancy, the transmission of sexually transmissible infections, and feeling bad about themselves. Parents will be shocked when they learn their child is involved in such activity. It needs to be handled sensitively. Children may feel guilty and blame themselves for ending up in this situation. Refer to Chapter 18 for information on what to do if this happens to your child.

Young people need to have the confidence to enjoy early sexual feelings without going on to have sexual intercourse. Sexuality education at puberty will help them gain this confidence. Ask your school about the sexuality education they provide and what you can do to support it.

Consider joining the Parent Teachers Association, community groups, health organisations or putting your name forward for the school board. You may be in a position to develop policies that address sexuality issues. Becoming involved in improving sexuality education at school or helping develop youth friendly services in the community is a great way to help all children.

Preparing for the future

Talking to your child about friendships, sex and relationships is important at this time. Talk about the basics of contraception, safer sex, signs of pregnancy, pregnancy options and the local health services available to young people. It is better to give children information before they become sexually active. Encourage them to think about the decisions they will need to make in the future. Research shows that young people who have had the opportunity to learn about these issues are more likely to delay sexual intercourse.[23]

Delaying intercourse will allow them to enjoy early sexual experiences such as kissing, touching and getting to know each other before making the decision to have sex. If they wait until they feel ready to take this step they are more likely to practise safer sex. Family Planning organisations and government agencies have pamphlets and websites with information that will update you on these topics.

Try these with your 9 – 12-year-old

- Ride through the moody times knowing that they won't last forever, and be patient through the times of high excitement. Children have as much difficulty being rational and making decisions when they are excited as when they are upset.
- Use everyday opportunities to talk about sex in an informal way.
- Encourage a healthy lifestyle by modelling a healthy lifestyle yourself and setting a good example.
- Get to know their friends, stay in touch with the music they like and what they like to do.
- Allow your child to make decisions and support them in the decisions they make.
- If your child has a disability allow them to take the same risks as other children.
- Work through an 'Online Safety Agreement' together. These give guidelines for the safe use of the net and are published by government and other agencies.[24]

Ask Me Anything

What *Ask me anything* is about

This part of *From Birth to Puberty* reviews ideas and skills that help in communicating values, feelings and information about sex and sexuality to young children. We've called it *Ask me anything* because we want you to be open, honest and available to communicate with your child. Tell them that you will try to answer all of their questions, and that you are happy when they come to you with questions.

There are three chapters in *Ask me anything*. Chapter 11 concentrates on the general principles parents should understand to develop an open, honest communication pattern that will help prepare young children for the changes ahead and for future relationships. Chapter 12 gives examples of how to answer your child's questions about sex and sexuality. Chapter 13 focuses on values, attitudes and sexuality. The examples are not to be taken as the 'correct' or 'right' or 'only' approach. You should apply and adapt them to your circumstances, as every family is unique.

11

Communicating with your child about sex

Two scenes from the home of the Jones family:

One morning in bed while passionately making love, Rita looked over Ben's shoulder, and standing in the open doorway was their four-year-old daughter Karly. Rita and Ben did not know how long she had been there. Rita hastily pulled away from Ben and sheepishly gave Karly her attention, as if nothing had been happening.

Later, Rita walked into the lounge with Karly's grandmother and found her three-year-old son Jake sitting in front of the TV playing with his penis. Rita desperately tried to divert grandmother's attention to the new pot-plant, while telling Jake to put his toys away!

Have you experienced something like this? Let's face it, family scenes like these involving sexuality are common. How you react in these situations shapes your child's attitude toward sexuality. Children learn as much or more from your emotional reactions as they do from what you say. Rita's reaction to these incidents sent her children a message about sexuality. If you find yourself over-reacting like Rita, you give the incident greater importance than it deserves. If you appear to treat sex as embarrassing, dirty or naughty, that is the message your child is receiving about sex. Children deserve to feel confident and enjoy their sexuality. Give them positive messages about sexuality so they go on to be confident, loving, caring adults and form healthy relationships.

What you think and feel about children's sexuality has a strong influence on how you respond to your child's sexual behaviour. Your experience of sexuality as a child, what your own parents said and did, your religious beliefs and cultural background, all contribute. Responding to your child in an open honest way will help them feel good about their sexuality. You risk making them feel ashamed, guilty or bad by responding to them in a negative way, or showing that you are not willing to talk about sexuality issues.

How difficult can it be?

I was doing the dishes with my seven-year-old grandson when he asked me what a boner was. I nearly dropped the plate. It flashed through my mind to tell him to wait until his mother came home, or not to be rude, or pretend that I didn't hear him. I managed to say, 'It's when your penis gets hard.' 'Oh', he said and started chatting about something else.

-Joanna, who was caring for her grandson

You may feel uncomfortable talking about sex with your child. Maybe you are uncertain how best to approach the topic. Discussing the subject comfortably need not be difficult. Knowledge of the basic facts of sexuality helps, but is less important than beginning open and positive communication at an early age. By showing a positive attitude toward sex and sexuality you will help your child feel more positive and confident.

106

Why do parents find talking about sexuality with their children so difficult? There are two main reasons. First, because sexuality is so personal. Most of us have grown up learning that our sexuality is a private matter, and this attitude persists when we come to talk to our own children.

Second, adults often have a view of sexuality that is associated with the physical side of sex. If we as parents project this adult view of sexuality onto children, we feel a dilemma.

> *It's all very well to talk about adults having sexual feelings,*
> *but children don't have sexual feelings do they?*
>
> -Ray, father of 2 girls

Like Ray, you may overlook the fact that all children, even as babies, are sexual beings. You may feel that if you acknowledge to your child that they have sexual sensations, then they may want to act on this in an adult way. You may think it inappropriate for innocent young children to be told about sex. If this is the case, your child will hear the message that sex is secret, that adults do not discuss it openly, if at all, when children are around.

One way to have a more relaxed approach is to decide in advance just what messages about sexuality you want to give your child and then to practice responding to anticipated questions and behaviour. By thinking ahead and taking the time to consider the underlying message that you are giving, you will find that your response is easier to make, and that it represents what you want to say. That's all very well, but how are you going to do that?

Talk with another adult

Talking about possible situations with your spouse, partner, or another friend can be helpful. To begin with, talk about how you learnt about sex, and how it was for you when you wanted to ask questions. Who did you ask? Who wouldn't you ask? Why?

Share your values and beliefs and why you feel the way you do about issues such as: sex on TV, breast-feeding in public, teenagers having babies, changing roles of men and women, sexuality education, soft porn magazines, sex outside of marriage. As you begin to feel more comfortable discussing these issues with another adult, you will become more confident tackling the simpler topics raised by your child.

If both parents have similar values and attitudes you will both give the same messages in response to your child's questions and behaviours. However it is unlikely that you and your spouse or partner are going to have the same values and attitudes on every aspect of sexuality. This won't be a problem if you both accept that you have differences, and respect each other's values. It is healthy for children to grow up in an environment where different values are expressed, as long as there is acceptance and respect of the differences. Issues involving differences in values, attitudes and sexuality are dealt with in Chapter 13.

Sending and receiving messages

In *Getting started* we stressed the importance of the messages you give your child. From a very young age, your child receives verbal and nonverbal messages about sexuality from you. The messages you give them in their early years are very significant and have a lasting impact. You start giving messages about sexuality from the time they are born. Although you can't have a conversation, you talk to your baby and communicate non-verbally in ways that help shape their sexuality.

You may respond emotionally to sexuality issues involving your child and later regret the messages that you sent. Those 'automatic' emotional responses may convey the same negative messages your own parents gave you in your youth. To avoid this, open and positive communication between you and your child should begin as early as possible, setting a pattern for effective future talks during adolescence and young adulthood. An advantage of talking about sexuality at a young age is that it is well before the hormonal changes of puberty affect children's thoughts and feelings about sexuality. It is also before your concerns become focused on the reproductive aspects of your child's sexuality.

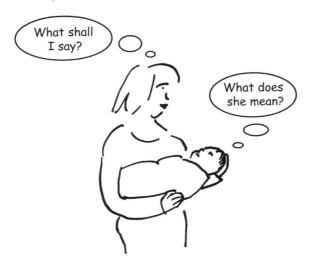

Mixed messages

Parents can easily give mixed messages about sexuality to their child. One parent sends a certain message and the other parent gives a conflicting one. Understanding and working through differences will help to avoid this and help you give clear messages to your child.

Marla is nine years old and wants to start shaving her legs, like the other girls at school. Her mother disagrees, telling her she is too young and could cut herself. She tells her that she didn't start shaving her legs until she had left school. Marla goes to see her father and asks if she could have one of his razors to shave her legs. He gives her one without a second thought.

Incidents like this can cause conflict between parents, simply because they had not discussed the issue before it arose. If you are alert to such situations and consult each other before making decisions, one parent will not feel that their wishes or their authority is being undermined.

Often your own parents or in-laws have strong feelings about sexuality issues and about the messages that children should be given. These can be quite different and perhaps at odds with your own. It may also become an issue with neighbours and friends if you help each other out with childcare. Having clearly decided on the messages you want to give your child provides you with the strength and confidence necessary to respond with conviction to concerned friends and relatives. If your child attends daycare you can also ask about their policies on issues such as privacy, nudity and sex play.

Use simple language and give facts

When talking to your child use simple language, and if you feel embarrassed or don't know the answer, say so. Children will understand how you're feeling. They will see that it's okay for them to ask questions, even if they are embarrassing.

Young children between 3 and 5 years old like basic factual information and are often satisfied with answers on that level[1]. Their questions are usually expressed in a matter-of-fact way.

> *Kylie (4 years) asked, "What's a tampon Mummy?" Diane showed her a tampon. "I see" said Kylie, and went off to play.*

What's a tampon?

Kylie's question was answered and she was satisfied knowing what the tampon looked like. Diane would probably have confused her daughter if she had started talking about periods and menstrual cycles when all Kylie wanted was to see a tampon. As children grow you will need different explanations of terms, to match their understanding at different ages. Older children and teenagers will ask more complex questions.

As adults we can easily read too much into young children's questions or comments, and try to probe or analyse their feelings. Young children find it difficult to talk about feelings. From about five years of age you can encourage them to say how they feel, and it will give them the confidence to recognise and express their feelings. Be careful not to divide their feelings into 'right' or 'wrong', or 'good' or 'bad', as children can end up doubting themselves.

Small children perceive, understand, and experience their world in a different way to adults. You need to understand this when deciding how to respond to your child's behaviour and questions. They generally have a very literal understanding of things and have difficulty comprehending abstract concepts. For example, when a child is told that a baby grows in mother's 'tummy', they may believe that the baby is mixed in with the food in her stomach.[2] So give basic information readily and address any misunderstandings your child may have. You will be laying the foundation for open, honest communication as your child develops.

Listen to your child

I happened to be passing the kid's bedroom when I overheard my 4-year-old James saying to his friend who had come over to play, "Give me a blowjob." I couldn't believe my ears. After listening and watching them for a while I realised they didn't know what it meant.

What would you do if your son said that? Before you say anything to your son, think. Children use sexual words in ways that make it seem they know more than they really do. A preschooler who says, "give me a blowjob" may just be repeating a phrase heard from adolescent brothers or sisters, with no understanding of the meaning of the words. If you respond negatively to this because you think he is being rude, your son will be confused because he does not understand the meaning of what he has said. Incidents like this can be a block to developing good communication. If it occurs regularly your child may become wary of speaking openly with you for fear of your reaction.

Listening and observing is more important than responding immediately. Delaying your response will give you time to think about what to say. If you overhear your 4-year-old James saying, "Give me a blowjob" to another child, neither of them is likely to know what it means. James is probably trying to sound clever, knowing his friend won't know what it means either. You could say, "Don't talk like that to your friend. I don't want to hear you use those words". You haven't had to explain what blowjob means but you have given a clear message that you don't want your child to use the term.

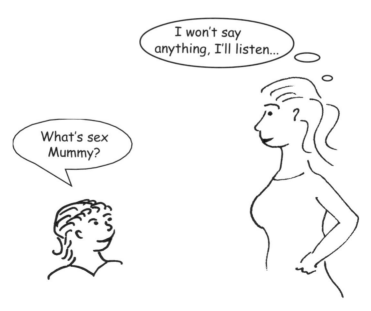

Good listening

Children learn to be good listeners when they have good role models. Listening is difficult. You think faster than you can speak and while someone is talking you are likely to be thinking about what you will say next rather than attending to what they are saying. It is also more than just listening to the words, because people communicate in other ways besides talking. Even if we do not respond verbally to a situation, our facial expression and body language can give a strong message. Be aware of the following non-verbal ways you and your child communicate:

- *Facial expressions*: raising eyebrows, smiling, frowning.
- *Body language*: nodding head, crossing arms, shrugging shoulders, looking away.
- *Tone of voice*: loud or soft, sad, excited – the feeling behind the words.[3]

When you are listening to your child, notice if what they say matches their tone of voice. If your child says, "I'm okay." in an unhappy voice, you will pick up the mixed message.

Here are some ways you can practise to become a good listener.

- If your child is upset and trying to express their feelings be silent as much as possible. Say things like "I see" or "really" so they know you are still listening.

- Show that you've heard and understood by reflecting the child's feelings back to them. For example, if your child says in an angry voice "I can't do this. I've tried and tried and it's too hard." A reply that shows you've heard their frustration would be "I can see that you're upset."

- Ask questions about what happened to make sure you've understood properly. Check that you have understood correctly by summarising what you have heard. For example, "You are upset because you have been trying for ages, and that wheel won't turn, right?"

- After the age of five encourage your child to talk about how they feel. You could say, "You look like you are getting very frustrated" or "You look a bit sad today". You will be helping them to express their feelings. By being a better listener you can pick up the emotion behind what your child is saying. Let them know you understand how they are feeling.

Be Positive

Giving your child attention in the form of encouragement, praise, smiles or cuddles, is a means of increasing a child's confidence in themselves. Show your child how to show affection by the way you treat them and by playing with their toys and pets. For example, you might praise them for showing affection to their little brother or sister, for being gentle with the neighbour's cat or expressing their feelings when playing with their teddy bear.

Remember when talking to children about acceptable behaviour, that they learn their most important and long- term lessons from *how* you say it[4]. So if your four year old walks into your bedroom when you are making love, explain to them that Mummy and Daddy are having a private cuddle and need to be on their own for a while. And what about grandma finding your son masturbating? It's normal, pleasurable behaviour, but it's something we do in private. Tell him,

> *Rubbing your penis is something you do in private, so you can do that in your bedroom, which is a private place. You don't do that in front of other people.*

114

This will let him know that there's nothing wrong with what he's doing, but that it will embarrass other people if he does it when they're around. If you are anxious about talking with your child about sensitive subjects, rehearse the words and the subject matter beforehand.

As they learn and grow, young children constantly repeat activities and questions. So in the early years you have many opportunities to give your child an understanding of the broad role sexuality plays in our lives. They learn about sexuality from observing you. They observe how you relate to others, how you express loving feelings, how you respect other peoples' differences including different values. If you would like your child to come to you for support when they are teenagers you need to start developing good communication when they are little. A comfortable pattern of communication will be established between you and your child - one that can extend into the teen years.

12

What to say and what to do

Suzie asked her father, "What's a virgin?" Her father said, "Ask your mother." Her mother said, "Don't they teach you that at school?" Suzie felt she was getting the run-around. She had a suspicion that if she put the question to her teacher she would be told to ask the school nurse or counsellor.

Almost every parent finds it hard to talk to their child about sex. We don't get much practice talking about it, and often our parents weren't very good at talking about it either. This chapter gives you examples, techniques and exercises to help you hone your skills. There is no 'right' or 'correct' way to respond to your child. No method works all the time and what works with one child may not work with another. So take the examples presented here as guides. Apply and adapt them. Don't be hung up on method or technique, the best thing you can do for your child is to respond in a positive manner to their questions and behaviours.

When should I start talking to my child about sexuality?

Start talking to your baby, using the 'proper' words for penis or vulva and vagina, when they are only a few weeks old. Use the words just as you would when talking to them about other parts of their body. Of course at this age your baby won't understand the words. However, talking to your baby using the 'proper' language is a useful rehearsal for later conversations. This is especially helpful for parents who are not comfortable using these terms for the genitals. Doing this will build confidence in your ability to talk about sexuality and you will be ready when your child is able to understand.

From the time your child is a toddler, opportunities to have talks about sexuality will arise naturally. Your child's curiosity can be used as a cue to provide information. For instance, when they comment about a pregnant woman, a sexual joke, or nudity, you can use this to open a conversation while they are interested. At these times they are more likely to talk and share their ideas, and listen to your ideas. So don't let these opportunities slip by – use them in preference to approaching the topic cold.

> *I was an orphan and went to a convent school. We had almost no sex education, and the nuns were incredibly modest. When I had my first child I was still ignorant of most of the correct words for the private parts, and had only a basic understanding of reproduction. I decided I would not let that happen to my children.*
>
> -Theresa, mother of four

Ideally by the age of 8 years you will have talked with your child about the changes puberty has ahead for them. This is especially important if they are an early developer and are entering puberty prematurely. If your child does not ask specific questions by age 7 or 8, open it up for them. Start by wondering out loud what you think they want to ask. Then wait. Rather than answering your question yourself, give them plenty of time to put it into their own words, to talk, to wonder, to think, and ask their own questions.

Talking and answering questions about sexuality

By talking to your child about their body and how they are feeling, they learn that it is okay to talk about these things. This will make it easier to talk about sexuality issues in the future. Answer your child's questions naturally so they learn they can ask you anything. Here are some tips to keep in mind:

- For young children, remember that as well as using simple language, the information or explanation should be kept simple.

- If you feel anxious or are not sure how to answer a question, it is better to delay your answer until you are happy with your response. Show that you are willing to discuss it at a better time by saying something like, "I can't answer that right now, let's talk about it tonight".

- Listen carefully to what they are asking or how they respond to you. Let them ask questions without interruption.

- Pay attention to your tone of voice. Keep it at the same level as your child's. If you raise your voice or are anxious, the meaning of your words will be swamped by the emotional message you are sending.

- Keep your answers brief. Give the information they are asking for, but don't extend your answer in great detail. Remember four-year-old Kylie from the last chapter? She asked, "what's a tampon?" and was satisfied when see saw one. If she wants more information she will ask for it, and you can continue the conversation.

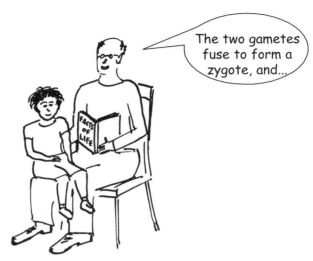

A 3 step process

Here is a process you can use to help work out a response to your child's question or behaviour. This 3 step process is a 'bare bones' approach, which we like for its simplicity.[5]

Step 1. *Think about why the child is asking the question or why they may be behaving this way.*
Step 2. *Decide what messages and/or information you want to give.*
Step 3. *Respond.*

Behaviour example

> *Gemma, age 6, had her friend Melissa home to play. Gemma's mother Brenda became suspicious when she saw they had closed the bedroom door for the third time. She opened the door and found them both hidden under a sheet with a torch, and their clothes scattered around the room. She realised they were exploring their bodies with the torch. She asked what they were doing and they sheepishly peeped out and said, "Nothing."*

Brenda took a breath and thought, "How shall I handle this?"
She thought (Step 1), "Why are they doing this?" They want
to see what they look like and to see if they look the same.
Then (Step 2), "What message do I want to give them?" She
wants them not to be secretive about what they are doing
and to know that they are not in trouble. She realises they
have been playing this game often and wants to make sure
they are both safe.
Response (Step 3). She says, "Are you both happy playing
this game or would you like to come with me and I'll read
you a story?"

Gemma and Melissa knew by the tone of Brenda's voice that they were not in trouble because of their game. By giving them a choice Brenda made it easy for either of them to stop the game if they were uncomfortable. She had suggested something else they could do.

Question example

Mark, age 7, asked his father Gary what periods are.

Step 1. *Why is Mark asking?*
He may have heard his mother or others talking about periods.

Step 2. *What messages and information does Gary want to give?*
Gary thought that Mark was old enough to understand the basic facts about periods. He wanted him to know that he was pleased that he asked.

Step 3. *Respond.*
Here is their conversation:

Mark: *What are periods?*

Gary: *A period is something women get for four or five days every month. A trickle of blood comes from their vagina.*

Mark: *Why does it happen?*

Gary: *Every month a woman's body gets ready to make a baby. Most of the time she doesn't make a baby, so she has a period.*

Mark: *Does it hurt?*

Gary: *It doesn't hurt like it does if you cut yourself and bleed. But some women get a stomach ache.*

Gary has responded to Mark's questions in a simple factual way with answers that Mark can understand. He doesn't need to go into details of the pain some women have with their periods. If you don't feel as confident as Gary in responding to a particular question you could read a book together. Check the book first to see that it is at a level your child can understand, and that you are comfortable with it. Stop reading when they are tired and let them pick it up later if they are interested.

Examples of responses to questions and difficult behaviours

Here are some examples of typical questions and behaviours from children three to twelve years old. The 3 step method is used with each example, showing how you could respond in these or similar situations. If the time is right you can encourage your child to continue talking. Some of these example responses end with a question and this is a good way to extend the talk.

3 year old daughter: "Let me feel your booboo (breast)."

1. She has seen me breastfeeding and sees her baby brother touching my breast and wants to find out what it feels like.
2. I want her to know that my breast is private and that I will put limits on her touching me. However it is not inappropriate for her to see what it feels like.
3. Response: *"My breast is a private part of my body. I don't want you to touch my breast now. You can see what it feels like when I'm feeding the baby after dinner if you like."*

5 year old daughter: "Mummy I don't like John. I want Daddy back."

1. She is probably missing her Dad and would rather see him at home than my new partner John.
2. She is sounding unhappy so I will respond to how she is feeling rather than to try to convince her that John is a nicer guy than her Dad.
3. Response: *"You sound sad. Are you missing Daddy? Shall we phone him and see if he can see you soon?"*

6 year old son: "Mummy what is this?" (child holding a tampon)

1. He is asking because he has found a packet of tampons in the bathroom and is curious to know what he has found.
2. He needs to know they are tampons. He is old enough to know something about periods. I want him to know I am comfortable for him to ask me about this.
3. Response: *"It's a tampon. I use them when I have my period. A period is something all women get so they can have babies."*

6 year old son. You are walking in the park and see two men kissing. Your son says, "Ooo look Mum, they must be faggots."

1. He has heard others talk about gay men in a negative way and he thinks it's okay to put them down.
2. I want him to know that gay men are the same as other men and that it is rude to put people down.
3. Response: *"They may be gay but it is rude to call anyone names whether they are gay or not. What do you know about men who are gay?"*

9 year old son: "Why aren't you on the pill?"

1. He may be wondering if we are planning to have more children or may be curious to know about other forms of contraception.
2. He knows that some women take The Pill but he may not know why. He is old enough to know about contraception. I want him to know I am comfortable for him to ask me about this.
3. Response: *"Taking the Pill is one way to stop getting pregnant. It is called contraception. Your father has had a vasectomy, which is another form of contraception. So we won't be having any more children."*

10 year old daughter: "What have periods got to do with sex?"

1. We have talked about periods but haven't really talked about sex. She is wondering how they are related and may want to find out if I am comfortable talking about sex with her.
2. This is an opportunity to open up a discussion about sex. I want her to know I am comfortable talking about this.
3. Response: *"A woman has a period so she can have a baby. To start a baby a man and a woman have sex. So really the two are related because they are both needed to have a baby. Do you want to ask me some questions about sex?"*

11 & 12 year olds.

Try rehearsing answers to these questions. They are questions young people of this age placed in an anonymous question box at school during a health course. You may recognise them from Chapter 10. Think about how you would respond to questions like these, before your child asks.

When is the right time to have sex?

Why do people kiss?

Does it hurt when a boy puts his dick up a girl's fanny?

Is sex dirty?

How would you know what hole to put it in?

Can you get stuck in the vagina?

What is a blowjob?

Is it okay to have sex at a young age?

You might feel uncomfortable about the language and content of these and other questions your child may ask. Separate the question from the way it is asked. Once you've done this, you can respond with language you feel is more appropriate. You will be modelling the language you want your child to use.

What if you've left it a bit late?

You've been hoping your child will ask questions and open up the conversation about sex themselves. But they haven't. And you have been putting it off. Does this sound like you? Don't worry, it's never too late. If you are in this situation, start now. Admit to your child that you want to have an important talk with them and you've been putting it off. Tell them why. It may be that you thought the school or their other parent would do it. You may have felt embarrassed, or not sure they were ready or how they would react. Follow this by telling them what you want to talk about. Using TV programs, books, magazine articles and current events is a good way to start a talk.

Here are some examples of how you could begin:

> *I want to talk about the changes that happen when you start puberty.*

> *I want to tell you what I think about teenagers starting to experiment with sex too early.*

> *I want to suggest what you could do if you were under pressure from your friends.*

Those examples all approach the topic directly. An alternative is to set a scenario to start the conversation:

> *Two friends were talking. One told the other they had done something bad and asked them not to tell anyone. Should the friend keep the secret?*

> *A group of 12-year-olds were going to a movie. One said 'I bet we could get into that R16 sex movie, let's go see it.' What would the others think about that?*

> *If a girl was going out with a guy and then found that he was two-timing, what could she do? How would she be feeling?*

These scenarios are ways to start talks about values and sexuality with your child. We explore this further in the next chapter.

We have reviewed the principles of good communication with young children, and given tips and techniques for talking with your child and answering their questions about sex. There are many good resources on communication skills and talking with your child about sex. Check your library, bookstore or the Internet. There is a list of resources under *Further Reading* at the end of this book.

13

Values, attitudes and sexuality

I always stopped Sally interrupting Ben and I when we were having a conversation and she wanted to ask something. "Wait until your father and I have finished talking, then you can ask your question," I said. I later thought how much I sounded like my own mother and how I was unaware that I had picked this up from her.

- Jane, talking about her 4-year-old daughter Sally

My mother taught me that it was wrong for me to wear clothes that revealed my breasts. I was shocked when Kelly wanted to wear fashionable tight-fitting singlet tops that revealed her early breast development. When I refused to allow Kelly to go to the movies in a singlet top it caused a major drama. I told Kelly she looked like a slut. I later felt terrible and wondered what had caused my outburst.

-Maxine, mother of 10-year-old Kelly

In both of these family stories the mothers, Jane and Maxine, were expressing a value they had acquired as children from their own mothers. We all form values at a very young age. Although we are not often consciously aware of them, they affect the way we relate to ourselves and to others. In Jane's case the value she expressed was that children should not interrupt when their parents are talking. Although Jane later realised that this value came from her mother, at the time her response to Sally was automatic.

Maxine was also expressing a value she had acquired as a child from her mother. Her mother had put a high value on modesty, and Maxine had in turn conveyed this in her reaction to her own daughter. Sometimes, because of your values, you put high or unrealistic expectations on yourself and on others. When these expectations are not reached you may judge other people unreasonably, as Maxine did in her outburst to Kelly.

You may have had negative personal experiences that make some situations involving your child difficult to respond to in a rational way. Trying to enforce your personal values on them rarely improves the relationship, and can lead to resentment and hostility. There are healthier ways to influence your child's values.

Values

Values are the rules we all have about how to behave. They are the accepted standards of a person or group. We learn them as we grow up, they form part of our belief system, and they influence our behaviour throughout life. Your values differ from other peoples depending on factors such as age, the family and society in which you grew up, school and other experiences. Most people have underlying values formed when they were young children. Although these values may change in adult life it usually takes years to do this.

Like everyone, you have your own package of values, attitudes and beliefs. They are part of who you are. They provide a framework that you use as you make decisions and live your life. In this chapter we look at how values about sexuality are expressed, how your values influence your child, and how you can help your child develop their own positive and healthy values.

Parents naturally want to encourage certain values in their children. You can promote your values in the belief that you know which values are desirable and what is right for your child. As in the stories at the beginning of this chapter, values are mostly taught by example. For instance, almost all parents would agree that honesty and respect are important ingredients in a healthy relationship. If you practise these values, you show your child how important these values are to you.

Differences in values

Within a family, parents may differ in some of their values, such as whether it is acceptable to be naked in front of the children, whether masturbation is normal, and in attitudes toward homosexuality. The following stories highlight some of the issues.

Brian enjoyed swimming naked in the family pool, which could not be seen by the neighbours. His wife, Jenny, objected to him doing this when their children were school age. Jenny and Brian talked about it many times, often in front of the children. Brian continued to do it, arguing that it was a perfectly natural thing to do. It was a worry to Jenny every summer for years, until Brian stopped when their daughter turned twelve.

Margaret (a European New Zealander) asked her daughter Puti (11 years) why she hadn't washed her hair when she had a shower. Puti said her Nanny (her Maori grandmother) had told her she should never wash her hair while she had her mate (period). Margaret thought that was ridiculous. "What's this stupid thing Nanny is telling you Puti? What right has she to tell my daughter this sort of rubbish?"

Tammy found one of the difficulties in her marriage with Hone was the way his whanau (family) treated their place as their own. Uncles, cousins and people she didn't even know would turn up for a meal unexpectedly, borrow their tools and never return them, or just hang out drinking their beer. But what really irritated her was how they assumed it was okay to call in and take her children to the river or out visiting without asking her or Hone.

The children in these stories are receiving different messages about values from their parents, grandparents or other relatives. The last two stories highlight value differences within families when parents come from different cultural backgrounds. There can be many differences in values between parents, including:

- The values, attitudes and beliefs about family, health, education, discipline and honesty.
- The way sexuality is expressed. For example, whether it continues to be appropriate to hug your son when he has reached puberty.
- The parents' experience of different role models (especially their own mother and father).
- The traditions, rituals and behaviours that are part of the parents' culture. Usually these have been handed down through many generations.

These differences can cause confusion for children if it involves conflict between parents about who is right or wrong. For example:

Don't listen to your Dad he doesn't know what he's talking about.

How can you avoid confusing your child with conflicting messages? How can you positively influence the values of your child and help them to decide for themselves what their personal values will be?

Clarify your values

Firstly, you need to be aware of how you as parents feel about different issues, by either discussing them with each other or with other adults. How do you feel about children exploring their sexual differences, teenage pregnancy, pornography or abortion? Do you think it's okay for your young son to wear a dress and lipstick when playing with the dress-up clothes at his pre-school? Do you think that it's okay for young children to run and play naked through the garden sprinkler outside on a hot day?

You may discover you are ambivalent or unclear about what you think is best for your child. Feeling uncomfortable is a sign that one of your strong values may be involved. You can check this by asking yourself if you are using words like 'should', 'must', 'never' or 'always'. These words are used to express deeply held values.

What if parents have different values? What can you do? Remember you or your partner may be unaware you are defending a strong value when you respond emotionally to a remark or behaviour. Accept that you do have differences and acknowledge the other's feelings. If you recognise that one or both of you are agitated, say something like:

> *We both seem to be getting upset, this must be something important.*

This shows acceptance and is likely to help. Acknowledging each other's feelings will help calm things down. Now talk it over, respecting each other's values. Talking it over will help you consider each other's perspective. If in the end you don't agree, this is not going to be a problem for your child. It is healthy for children to grow up in an environment where different values are expressed, as long as there is acceptance and respect of the differences.

Values and beliefs

For most people values and beliefs mean the same thing. However they are given different meanings by academics. Beliefs are principles or propositions that we accept as true, often without proof. Examples are religious faith and spiritual beliefs. Values can usually be distinguished from beliefs because values contain a moral judgement about what people 'should', 'ought', 'must', or 'always' do.[6] The implication is that people are 'wrong' or 'bad' if they don't behave in that way. For example, I may have a value that parents 'ought' not be seen naked in front of the children. I would judge people who allowed their children to see them naked as not reaching my standards. Values also have varying degrees of strength, ranging from little importance to most important. A very strong value would be based on the message "parents *must never* be seen naked by the children".

Helping shape your child's values

Talking to your child about your values and beliefs and why you hold them will help them to understand your point of view and to form their own values. You can acknowledge that other people will not necessarily think the same way as you. You will help your child to be less judgmental of others by showing you respect other people's values and that you do not expect everyone to have the same beliefs as you. By doing this you also show your child they are free to question and talk openly and honestly about sexuality issues with you. Like you, they can explore and assess their own attitudes in order to develop their own values. They will develop insights into how they relate to others. When your child is clear about what they value they will be able to make healthier decisions, and initiate actions based on those values.

How do you help your child develop these skills? Respect for themselves and others will develop if you show your child that you believe in these values yourself. They will find it easier if your own behaviour reflects your values. Try to 'walk the talk'. Your child will be watching you closely and will be your greatest critic. If you value honesty and openness in a relationship be sure you treat your partner in this way. If you believe people should be treated with respect be sure you treat your child with respect.

Take an interest in their friends and their interests. Be available to respond to their requests for help and support. Valuing their opinions and being positive about things they do well will build your child's self-esteem.

Self-esteem

Our self-esteem is the extent to which we value ourselves. Self-esteem is our basic frame of reference, and is largely formed through interaction with others during childhood. It influences how we perceive and interpret our relationships with other people. Children's self-esteem has a large bearing on how they accept and cope with their developing sexuality.

You can help your child develop their unique self and their self-esteem in many ways. The following list gives some examples of ways you can show respect for your child.

- Let them arrange their room as they wish
- Allow them to choose clothes they want to wear
- Respect their opinions and privacy
- Ask for their advice
- Show them you enjoy their company and like to have them around.
- Encourage them to display their paintings, constructions, or things they have found.

Giving respect and freedom of choice does not mean giving them a license to behave as they wish. Limits and ground rules must be set. Setting and maintaining these rules helps your child know what your values are, and also helps them establish their individuality. By developing your child's self-esteem you help them to be honest in their relationships and positive about their growing individuality.

Rules and moral development

Setting rules and limits to behaviour are necessary to preserve the innocence of your child. However rules learned as children can change and become inappropriate values as we grow older. For example, the childhood rule "I must never talk to strangers", may later be unconsciously broadened to become a value such as "I never trust people I don't know". This value is inappropriate in adult life. Introduce new rules to replace outdated ones as your child grows. Setting rules for a five-year-old is much easier than for a twelve-year-old. With an older child try negotiating a shared set of rules and writing them down.

Like other aspects of their growth, your child's moral standards – their sense of right and wrong, or ethical conduct - develop in stages through childhood. Different children progress at different rates. Toddlers decide if what they want to do is right or wrong by whether it will bring them pleasure or punishment. At the next stage children usually make decisions on ethical behaviour to meet the approval of their parents. Teachers and religious groups may also have an influence. It won't be until puberty or later that most children will be capable of basing their moral or ethical decisions on principles that they have accepted for themselves as true.[7]

Giving clear messages about what you think is right will help your child develop their own values and moral standards. They will hear that you can support your values with good arguments and will learn to do the same.

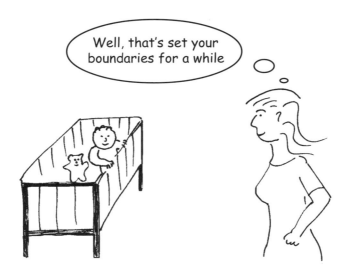

Values and decision-making

Dion and his wife Mary-Lou were having problems with their sex life. Mary-Lou suggested they attend counselling but at first Dion resisted this because he valued his privacy. He did not want to talk with a counsellor about their problems. On the other hand, he valued his relationship with Mary-Lou, and on reflection decided his relationship was more important than his privacy. They arranged an appointment with a counsellor.

We all make decisions based on our values. In the example above Dion held two competing values about counselling, one for and one against. He made his decision after considering which value he held most strongly.

In a similar way our children are often exposed to conflicting values from different people or groups of people. You can offer one set of shoulds and should-nots to your child and their peer group may offer another. For example, consider this situation:

> *Connie would not allow her daughter Anna (9 years) to wear make-up. "You're too young," she said. Anna thought that Connie was living in the dark ages because all her friends wore make-up.*

You may believe your daughter is too young to wear make-up, but if her peer group all wear it, she is likely to think her friends are doing the right thing. You need to consider this before making the decision to impose your own values. Often a compromise can be reached.

The messages young people receive about what are 'desirable' values are often inconsistent. Teachers, politicians, movie stars, music idols and religious groups all present different values and attitudes. Being unclear about what to believe and who is right can cause conflict and confusion for your child, especially when their parents' views differ from the views of their friends. Some young people will adopt their friends values and make decisions based on peer pressure. Some will adopt their parents values, and other will have a mix of their parents and peers values.

Sometimes lip service can be paid to the 'desirable' values of parents but the young person's behaviour contradicts these values. Many young people from age 9 or 10 say that they don't talk to their parents about what they are doing because they know their parents wouldn't approve. They would rather paint a rosy picture to keep the approval of their parents than to risk, in their eyes, losing their parents love. You can help avoid this situation with your own child by working to keep the communication channels open.

Attitudes

Ray reacts to gay men with derogatory comments. He advocates public policies against them, such as gay men should not be allowed to join the armed forces.

Ray has an unfavourable attitude toward gay men. He consistently judges all gay men as not worthy of the same rights as others.

Kathy consistently praises female artists, and regularly attends exhibitions of their work. She also buys paintings by female artists to hang in her apartment.

Kathy has a favourable attitude toward women's art. In these two examples we can see how an attitude can be observed from a person's behaviour. After observing someone behaving badly we may say, "Jimmy has an attitude" or "Tania has an attitude problem." However attitudes can be positive as well as negative.

Attitudes have been defined as our likes and dislikes, or our evaluation (judgement) of an event or people or objects. You tend to classify events, people and objects, and to judge them in a consistent way, as in Kathy's attitude to art, or Ray's attitude to gay men. Your attitudes are communicated to others through your behaviour. They show how you think and feel about something.

At a parent workshop Angela told other parents that when she breastfed her 4-month-old baby, her two-year-old son would tuck his teddy under his T-shirt and pretend to breastfeed him too. She wanted to know if that was normal behaviour. The other parents generally agreed that he was merely copying Angela and that it was nice to see him being so caring. Suddenly one of the fathers in the group burst out that he thought it was appalling, that if the boy were his son he would be disgusted and said he thought, "It would make the boy gay."

This father's reaction was emotional. His behaviour revealed the attitude he had toward homosexuality.

Attitudes and values

Attitudes are linked to values but they are not the same as values. Social psychologists have a number of ways of distinguishing attitudes from values. Most see values as very broad, whereas attitudes are narrow and relate to specific situations or events. This is the distinction used in this book. Here are some examples to help you distinguish attitudes from the underlying values:

I hate it when you don't close the bedroom door when you get changed. (attitude)
Parents should not be seen naked in front of the children.(value)

How can you suggest we go away for a weekend without the children. (attitude)
Children always come first. (value)

Stop fondling me in front of the children. (attitude)
Couples should not publicly display their affection. (value)

Opinion is another term used along with values and attitudes. Some social psychologists define this as being more specific than attitudes. An example of an opinion is:

I think Jennifer Lopez is better than Madonna.

-Jay, 11 years

Changing attitudes

Attitudes are more easily changed than values, and attitude changes are often associated with changes in life circumstances. For example, a man who said he would never marry again after his first marriage ended in divorce may change his attitude when a relationship later develops with a new partner. The attitudes that our children have about certain things are often different from those of their parents. A 9-year-old daughter may think that wearing make-up to the movies is a good idea, whereas her parents may not. Parents of young adolescents know that many arguments with their children are due to differences in attitudes.

> *I seem to have arguments now with Anna (13 years) over the smallest things, what food she will eat, what time she goes to bed, and now we have all the boyfriend issues to deal with.*
>
> -Carol, mother of Anna

Parents who have been together for some years often develop similar attitudes about sexuality and appropriate expressions of sexuality. They may have had different attitudes when they first met, influenced by their own family upbringing. However over time they often adapt their attitudes to accommodate each other. For new couples and the instant families created by stepfamilies, there has been no time to develop similar attitudes. These issues for stepfamilies are explored in Chapter 17.

Values, attitudes and family dynamics

David and Louise were very happy with the birth of Ben, their first child. Ben seemed to give them a common bond that made them feel more like a family. After a few weeks it became clear that David and Louise had different ideas about

139

parenting. David wanted Ben to be circumcised but Louise did not agree. David also wanted Louise to breastfeed Ben but after a few weeks Louise put him on the bottle.

David enjoyed feeding Ben in their bed when he woke at night, and wanted to let Ben stay in the bed and sleep as he cuddled him after his feed. However Louise insisted he put Ben back in his bassinette. David began to feel that he wasn't having any say in family decisions. He decided to do other things for himself outside the family.

When a couple have their first child the family dynamics change. The new parents may need to work through some of their values and attitudes to accommodate the baby. There are two important influences present in every family with two adults and one or more children: a 'togetherness tendency' that draws family members together; and the need for individuality or separateness of each family member. The challenge is to maintain a balance between the two influences.

Family togetherness

Family members tend to be drawn together. Part of this tendency is instinctive and is associated with early experiences of closeness and bonding to parents and family. We remember the feeling of security that this gave when we were young, it is something we value, and seek to provide as parents in our own families. This shared value acts as a bond between family members.

The other aspect of family life that binds members together is their shared emotional experience. This is the result of the emotions that family members experience in their relationships with each other. Over time these become habitual (learned) emotional responses, and may range from very pleasant to very unpleasant. Whether the emotional experience is positive or not, these emotions become automatic, and their familiarity helps bind people together. [8]

Individuality

The tendency for family togetherness exists alongside the need for individuality. Family members are very different from each other. They may not be aware of many of the differences, especially at the beginning of a marriage or partnership. When two people enter a relationship they are usually inclined to think they are similar, and of course this is often why they are attracted to each other in the first place. However some of the differences between partners can mean they will have different ideas about parenting, including what sexuality values they would like their children to adopt, and on how to communicate these values to their children.

In David and Louise's case, the differences over Ben led David to do more on his own, outside the family. He needed to have time out for himself. It was his way of trying to achieve a balance between his need for individuality and the need for family togetherness. He also had a need to feel that Louise valued his parenting views. Doing things individually is good for each parent's personal growth and while it develops individuality it needs to be balanced with doing things with the family. This will avoid developing isolation, which causes problems in a relationship.

Your child's need for individuality

Your child needs to maintain or achieve a sense of being a separate person. This begins to develop at an early age, as a two-year-olds tantrum demonstrates. A two-year-old will stand and demand, perform and cry, trying to get his or her own way. If you are always putting pressure on your child to be as you want them to be, they often rebel. A common reaction to you 'laying down the law' is that they will deliberately rebel to oppose your authority.

Sarah (9 years) said her mother told her she should always wash her hair once a week or it would fall out. So she didn't wash it for a month to see if her mother was right.

This kind of rebellion in children can be positive and healthy, although Sarah's example isn't very hygienic. The positive outcomes include the ability to think and speak for themselves, to respect the individuality of others and not try to make others conform to their own opinions or values.

The greater the pressures are for a family member to conform to the values or behaviours of other family members, the more likely it is that the person will resist and fight to be different.

> *Trevor used many swear words in conversation. His wife and his in-laws constantly asked him not to swear in front of the children. The more they nagged, the more he swore. It was a vicious cycle.*

Each of us is unique. We have genetic differences, different lessons learned from our families and communities, and different ways of coping with life. Your child is developing their own unique qualities, and you can help them by creating an emotionally healthy climate. As you clarify your values, and develop your communication and listening skills, you can model the behaviour you would like to see in your son or daughter.

Try these with your child

- Choose what you are going to make an issue of, and let other less important issues go. For example, you can emphasise cleanliness, but let your child dress the way they want. Concentrate on issues that affect the rest of the family, for example, the time they take in the shower.
- Talk about your expectations. For example, personal hygiene, helping around the home, TV viewing.
- Sit down together and work out chores that they can do: feeding the cat; emptying the garbage; changing their bed sheets.
- Set rules for hellos and goodbyes. For example, introducing their friends to you when they bring them home.
- Talk about the importance of trust and honesty. Use the scenario ideas from the last chapter to start the discussion.
- As your child gets older increase their responsibility for decision making. Show them how to break seemingly overwhelming decisions into meaningful parts. Express your confidence in their ability to make good decisions.[9]

At School

14

Sex education at primary school

"Do you want Mr Drysdale talking to Nadine about sex?"
Fran asks Nadine's mother Lucy anxiously.
"No, but I don't think they do that yet. But they do talk about
periods. Can you imagine him talking about periods? You
know what men are like," replied Lucy.
"Yeah I know and I don't think half the kids are ready for it.
They would have to separate the girls and boys wouldn't
they? Rawinia would be so embarrassed."
Soon twenty-five parents are sitting in rows at the front of
the school hall, waiting for the parent consultation meeting
to begin. Along with Lucy and Fran, they are wondering
how sex education classes will be handled and aren't sure
that they want their children to be involved.

Mention sex education to a parent whose child has just started primary
school and you are likely to draw a blank expression at best. When
your child starts school you will probably not have given a lot of
thought to the role the school will play in their sexuality education.
However, from the time they begin school they usually take part in a
health education program that includes a sexuality component.

Like Fran and Lucy, you may have concerns that the teachers will
be talking about such a personal subject and wonder if it is appropriate
for them to be discussing any aspect of sexuality. This chapter

addresses some of these concerns. It also explains how you can have input into the sexuality education program and gives a checklist of what a good program should contain.[1] These are the most asked questions from parents:

Isn't it my job to teach my child about sex?

Yes. Your child learns more from you than anyone. They learn about relationships and values and how to express their feelings from you. Many parents are wonderful teachers of sexuality, giving their children a strong sense of values and modelling healthy relationships. Some parents are comfortable talking about sexuality and some are not.

What can schools do that I can't?

Schools can complement your child's learning from home and provide social learning opportunities that are not possible within the family.[2] In the classroom children have the opportunity to practise communication skills. Young people are encouraged to be open and honest with each other when talking about sexuality issues. In the classroom children can hear each other's opinions and gain an understanding and tolerance of others. The school can give up-to-date, accurate information that is sometimes not easily accessible to parents. And your child has an opportunity to discuss matters with their teachers. This is different from discussing these matters with you, because teachers are not emotionally involved with them in the way you are as a parent.

> *Hinehou, a Maori community worker, was finding it difficult to talk to her daughter, Merita, about the changes she would be going through at puberty. When her daughter's school notified her that they would be discussing sexuality issues at school it motivated her to get started. She was surprised at how much Merita already knew, even though some of her*

ideas were confused. Hinehou was pleased she had been 'pushed into it' by the school, especially as Marita had her first period soon after.

While the program is on at school you can use the opportunity to talk to your child about sexuality. Ideally, you tell your child what to expect at puberty. However not all parents talk to their children and give them the information they need. Most boys in school sexuality courses say their parents don't talk to them about sex. Some girls are not prepared for puberty by their parents either.

When asked what she learnt from the course on puberty an 11-year-old girl wrote: "I learnt heaps, most things I wouldn't learn at home. I thought it would be shaming but it wasn't. I didn't even know about periods."

Talk to your child well before puberty about the changes ahead. Talk to them about your own values and the expectations you have of them. This will help them to develop their own set of values.

Will teaching my child about sex at primary school destroy their innocence?

No. Although children are given information on sex and sexual matters, they do not understand or act on it in the way adults do. Researchers argue that children's understanding is limited regardless of how much information they are given.[3] They can only learn what they are ready to learn. There is a large gap between children and adults in reasoning and comprehension. This gap protects young children's innocence and your child will not be corrupted or harmed by the information.

Children are naturally curious about issues relating to sexuality. They are exposed to many sexuality messages on television, through music and in magazines. They also hear negative things about sex, particularly sexual violence and rape. It is important to balance these messages with positive messages about sexuality, which is after all a natural part of our lives. Children learn maths, science and language from an early age, building on what they learn each year. The same principle applies to learning about their bodies and relationships.[4] Delaying the introduction of sexuality education and the biology of reproduction until your child is a teenager is too late. By that time sexual messages from the media and misinformation from peers and other sources may have lead to sexual experimentation and more serious consequences of sexual behaviour.

How do I have input into the school sexuality education program?

In New Zealand, parents are invited every two years to discuss and have input into their school's sexuality education program. The school will usually notify you through a newsletter or letter that a consultation meeting is to take place. The letter will include information about the proposed program. You can use this meeting to hear about the way the program has been put together, examine lesson plans, debate the underlying values of the program, to ask teachers questions about the program and to learn how you can support it. You are also given the option to remove your child from the class while the course is being taught.

> *Loleni, a Samoan mother of a very sexually mature 11-year-old daughter, said that she felt it was inappropriate for the school to be talking about sex to the children. She said that it went against her culture. However, when she learned the content of the program she was surprised that it was so comprehensive. She wanted her daughter to be included except for the lesson discussing sexual intercourse and sexual relationships. That was one lesson of the 14 lessons planned.*
> *After much discussion with the teacher, Loleni decided she*

would not remove her daughter for that lesson. She felt it would be impractical and could make her daughter feel that she was being treated differently from the rest of her class. The teacher explained that if she changed her mind she could always get in touch with the school and ask that her daughter be removed.

Parents are often surprised that the program is comprehensive and is not just talking about sex. In practice, few parents remove their children from sexuality classes.

Some schools invite you or other members of the family to participate in activities in some of the lessons. The way in which this opens up discussion between parents and their children can be striking.

An activity parents and children both enjoy is learning the correct terminology for the sexual and reproductive parts of the body. Each group of two or three is given a grid with names of parts of the body. They then match the words on the page with a simple description of that part. These descriptions are on separate cards.

When the task is complete the cards are turned over. If the words have been correctly matched the cards form a picture. The group can see where they may have made a mistake and learn from it. Both the parents and their children always enjoy this activity. They laugh together at their mistakes and eagerly try to work out where they have gone wrong. GL

How will I know if the school has a good sexuality education program?

A good sexuality education program gives you the chance to talk to the teachers about the topics to be covered and how the program will be run. The topics will be appropriate to the age of the children.

The program will reflect the cultural values of the school community.

Here is a checklist of what should be covered in a good program at the primary school level. You can compare this with the program offered by your school. The children should learn:

- to feel good about their sexuality
- appropriate ways to express their feelings
- to have an understanding about the reproductive and sexual parts of the body
- about the changes at puberty
- to be clear and strong in stating what they want and what they don't want
- what to think about when they make decisions
- ways to stand up to peer pressure
- how to discuss sexuality openly with their peers
- what to think about before having a sexual relationship
- about pregnancy and birth
- how to discuss sexuality with their parents

Do parents want primary schools to teach sexuality education?

Yes, almost all parents do support sexuality education at school. Parent surveys[5] show that the vast majority of parents support sexuality education in schools. Family Planning Association educators also find this to be the case in the schools they work in.

Sexuality educators know that a well-designed program has other positive results. At a parent consultation meeting at a school for children aged 10 to 12, the Principal stated that each year he never fails to be impressed by the way their sexuality education program changes the attitudes of the students. Instead of treating sexuality as secretive, naughty and rude, they develop a respectful and responsible attitude toward it.

Do teachers have adequate training in this area?

Some do and some don't. No teacher should be expected to teach a sexuality program unless they have had the training and the resources to do so competently.

When teachers begin teaching sexuality education they may feel anxious talking about such a personal topic. However, most teachers are surprised how comfortable they become once they get started. They find they relate to the students in a more personal way than they do when teaching more academic subjects.

> *During a teacher training course I facilitated, Wendy, a teacher of 10-12 year olds, couldn't imagine how she was going to explain sexual intercourse to her class. The teachers practised describing sexual intercourse during a role play activity. Wendy found that after three practices she was able to sound quite natural but wondered how easy it would be with her students. She rang me a few weeks later to report how pleased she was with the comfort she felt when the time came to talk to her class and she wondered why she had been so worried about it.* GL

From their training teachers realise that they do not need to be experts in sexuality. To deliver the course they should be comfortable discussing sexuality, be proficient at assisting the children to develop communication and relationship skills, and ensure that the information passed on is accurate. However, teachers will not have all the answers to children's questions. If they are not sure of the answer to a query they will work with the student to find an answer or in some cases refer the student back to the parent.

Will the teachers impose their own values on my child and undermine the values I want them to learn?

No. Teachers are trained to be clear about the difference between facts and opinion in their sexuality teaching. If they talk about opinions it will not be their personal opinions, it will be inclusive of a range of opinion. The role of sexuality education at primary school is to complement learning at home, not to challenge or undermine your values.

Will talking about sex encourage my child to experiment?

No. Students in these programs are more likely to delay having sex until they are older and they are less likely to get pregnant when they are teenagers.[6,7] Sexual behaviour will not be discussed at school until your child has reached the age of puberty. During these classes the teacher will give clear messages that it is best to delay sexual intercourse until they are older.

The students learn ways to resist pressure in sexual situations. Practising to respond assertively in role-plays in the classroom prepares them to resist pressure from their friends. Examples of role-play scenarios are: being pressured into lying to their parents; to be someone's boyfriend or girlfriend; or experimenting with sex.

A sample of comments made by 11 and 12-year-olds when asked what they had learnt from a sexuality course about sexual relationships were:

That you should think about everything before you rush in.

That having sex can cause heaps of problems and so it's better to wait.

That when we start having sex we should use protection if we don't want a baby.

That you can get pregnant the first time.

When asked if they thought they were too young for this information they made the following comments:

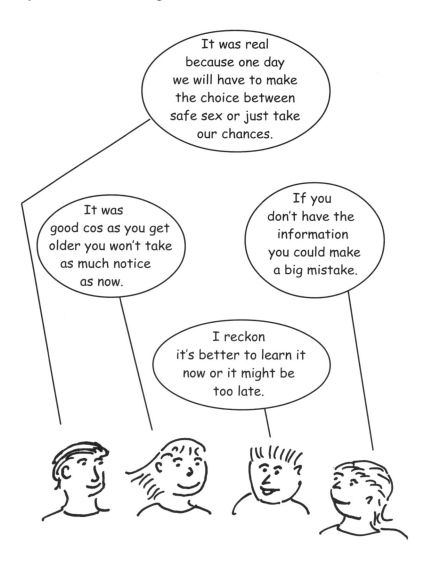

Isn't abstinence the best thing to teach my child?

Of course primary school children are too young to have sexual intercourse. Sexuality education programs at this level will give this message very clearly. Your first thought may be that teaching abstinence would seem to be the best approach to take with your child. And in fact abstaining from sex is the message that is clearly given by teachers. However, to some people abstinence means not just abstaining from sex, but the denial of any sexual feeling or sexual pleasure. Like other feelings, it is impossible for a child not to have these feelings.

Rejecting children's feelings and denying them all forms of sexual or sensual pleasure is inappropriate and can lead to secrecy and guilt. When you hear proponents argue their case for abstinence to be taught in your child's school, ask for the detail of what abstinence means in their proposal. Does it mean abstaining from all touching and kissing for example? Once you have this information you can make an informed decision.

Will the program teach my child that homosexuality is normal?

The program acknowledges the sexual diversity in the community and at the school. Schools do not tolerate discrimination of any kind and they will be inclusive of all sexual orientations in their teachings. Schools usually have policies that include the objective of enabling all students to reach their academic and social potential without prejudice. They can only do this if they seek to provide an environment that is inclusive and affirming of gay, lesbian and bisexual people in all aspects of school life. The majority of children at primary school will be unaware of their sexual orientation until they reach their teens. However, the primary school can play a part in developing non-discriminatory attitudes and dispel myths surrounding homosexuality.

Some people find it hard to acknowledge that homosexuality is a normal part of human sexuality. Some people feel it is acceptable to display negative attitudes to gays, lesbians and bisexuals. Parents may fear that schools are encouraging homosexuality. However a person's sexual orientation is a result of their natural attractions. A child can't catch homosexuality or be encouraged to be gay, nor can people have their sexual orientation changed.

You decide

The introduction of sexuality education programs in primary schools has been debated strongly, with some groups and individuals opposing it on the

Can I go to the sex classes at school?

grounds that it undermines family values. We believe you should be well informed about what these programs involve. You can then make up your own mind whether the program offered at your child's school is compatible with your views and values. In the next chapter, we review the content of a typical primary school sexuality course and give examples of activities your child will be involved in.

15

What will my child learn?

Sexuality education is a process, not a one-off talk with mum or dad, or one course at school. It begins in infancy and continues into adulthood. Your role as a parent is crucial and so is the collaboration between parents and the school to deliver appropriate and quality sexuality education. Your child will be learning aspects of their sexuality at school.

Educators recognise that sexuality education is a process that starts before children enter school, continues during school and after they leave. Schools aim to complement and build on the learning children have from home, in the wider social context that a school can offer. This chapter outlines the main topics in primary school sexuality education programs, so that you know how the school guides the process, and what your child will be learning.

The program

Sexuality education programs are designed to give the information and develop the skills needed to prepare your child for adulthood. Unlike the sex education classes of a decade ago, they do not only address the biological aspects of reproduction. They focus on helping young people feel good about who they are, giving them skills to have positive relationships with others, and helping them look after themselves.

Sexuality education seeks to assist children in understanding a positive view of sexuality, provide them with information and skills about taking care of their sexual health, and help them acquire skills to make decisions now and in the future.
-National Taskforce on Sexuality Education, USA[8]

The underlying principle in this approach to sexuality education is that everyone is important, unique and deserves respect. Each child will develop their sexuality at their own rate. The underlying values of the sexuality education program may include: a respect for other people and their individual differences; honesty; that sexuality is a natural and healthy part of who we are; that children will be given accurate factual information; and the value of developing and maintaining healthy relationships.

Different schools will run slightly different programs because each school can plan their own lessons. They are guided by the objectives in the curriculum and the needs of their students. In New Zealand, the Ministry of Education requires primary and secondary schools to include sexuality education as part of their health program, although in practice not all schools provide a comprehensive program at all levels.

Children enter school with varying levels of knowledge. They also have different experience of and comfort with talking about sexuality issues. Topics are introduced and then picked up and extended again later, at a level appropriate to their age and understanding. Reviewing and building on each topic in consecutive years addresses these differences between children.

Marea had a 9-year-old son, Jeff, who was very small for his age. The difference in physical maturity between Jeff and his friend Todd, also 9, was remarkable. Jeff looked like a child; Todd had the build of a young man. The school informed parents that their health program would be teaching about the changes at puberty. Marea could see that this was appropriate for Todd but was concerned her son would not be ready for it because it was obviously going to be some time before he reached puberty.

Children who are at Todd's level of maturity will find the information relevant. While it may not be relevant to Jeff at this time it will be reintroduced later and he will benefit from it then. Participating in the earlier lessons will not disadvantage Jeff and he can build on this introduction next time.

What is in a primary school sexuality education program?

A good example of the way schools may be guided in health and sexuality education is contained in The New Zealand Health and Physical Education Curriculum[9]. There are seven key areas of learning: mental health; sexuality education; food and nutrition; body care and physical safety; physical activity; sport studies; and outdoor education.

The sexuality education component requires students to develop communication skills, problem-solving skills, a respect for themselves and others, an understanding of their rights and responsibilities, and an understanding of sexual and reproductive development. It is based on the concept of well-being and the Maori concept hauora. Well-being encompasses the physical, mental and emotional, social, and spiritual dimensions of health.

Hauora is a philosophy of health unique to New Zealand. It comprises taha tinana (physical well-being), taha hinengaro (mental and emotional well-being), taha whanau (social well-being), and taha wairua (spiritual well-being). Teaching sexuality in the context of their social and emotional maturity as well as their physical maturity is recognised in this approach. The curriculum also requires the program to be appropriate to the age of the child and reflect the cultural values and the kaupapa (philosophy) of the school community.

Topics at each stage

Primary school - the first 3 years at school.

Children learn how their bodies work, the names for parts of their bodies including the sexual parts, the differences between male and female, and how to care for themselves. They learn to identify and talk about feelings, and to be assertive. They learn about friends and friendships, and how to ask for help if they don't feel safe.

Examples of what kids aged 5 to 7 do

1. *Body jigsaw.* The children assemble a life-size jigsaw of a child and place labels with the names of each part on the jigsaw. They discuss other names they know for each part (other languages or slang words).
2. *Feelings activity.* The teacher displays a photograph of children with different expressions and asks the children to identify their feelings. Each feeling is discussed using questions such as: How do you know the person is feeling this way? Why might they be feeling this way? In what situation might you be feeling this way? How would your body be feeling when you felt this way? The activity is repeated with different feelings - happy, sad, angry, worried, relaxed.

Ages 7 to 9.

At this level children learn about differences in families, caring for each other within the family, and about family break-ups. Pregnancy and birth are covered and managing difficult feelings. They practice communication skills, making decisions and managing the consequences of those decisions.

Examples of what kids aged 7 to 9 do

1. *Decision-making activity.* Small groups of students are each given a situation where a decision needs to be made, such as: a child has seen another take something out of someone else's school bag, or a child has been waiting for their parent to collect them and they haven't arrived. The students fill out a work sheet listing the possible actions that could be taken, the possible consequences for each action, and decide what they think the best action would be. They then present their findings to the class.

2. *The structure of families.* Students are given cards representing the people in one family. Another baby or child joins the family and the concept of adopting or fostering is discussed. They then imagine the parents are very unhappy with each other and decide to separate, even though they still love their children. The concepts of separation, divorce, and different custody arrangements are discussed. The possibility of different parents getting together to form a stepfamily is discussed.

Ages 10 to 12.

The program at this stage includes teaching about the physical and emotional changes at puberty, changing friendships and maintaining friendships. Students learn more about being assertive, making decisions and dealing with peer pressure. They examine gender roles, body image messages and the differences in family structures and values. They learn about expressing sexual feelings, sexual relationships and making decisions in a relationship.

Examples of what kids aged 10 to 12 do

1. *Changes at puberty.* The teacher has a container with changes at puberty written on individual pieces of paper and a poster of a

young woman and a young man. Students are asked to take one of the changes and decide if the change is relevant to boys or girls. The change is placed on the poster indicating if the change happens in boys, girls or in both. Each change is discussed. The changes include: breast development, hairy armpits, pimples, bigger muscles, larger penis, wet dreams, getting hungry often, etc. Discussions would include the fact that some boys get breast development at this time, what you can do about pimples, what wet dreams are and how to manage them.

2. *Choices and consequences.* Photos of teenagers and personal statements about their sexual situations are distributed to the class. The students read the statements and interpret the sexual decisions that the teenager has made to the rest of the class. Examples are:

Lucy: "When I was 15 I wanted to have sex to see what it felt like. I thought that since it was my first time I didn't have to worry. Boy was I wrong. I got pregnant."

James: "I hear others talking about sex. I wonder what it's like sometimes but I'm also scared. I don't think I'll do it 'til I've left school."

Maria: "No way am I ready to go all the way. There's no guy that I like in that special way. Besides, I've got plans for my life and a baby would really mess that up."

Through this activity students understand the choices and consequences involved in the decision to have intercourse or wait to have intercourse. They identify the choices that hypothetical teenagers have made. They also see that some decisions are more difficult than others.[10]

Do teachers notice changes in the children's behaviour following the program?

Yes. Teachers typically note three areas of behaviour change:

1. The children become more relaxed and confident to seek answers to their questions about sexuality.
2. They continue discussing issues about puberty and relationships after the course has ended and seek clarification of their ideas through talking with their teachers.
3. They have more respect for each other and become more mature in their attitudes. For example, the giggling and whispering about sexual matters is replaced by a willingness to talk openly.

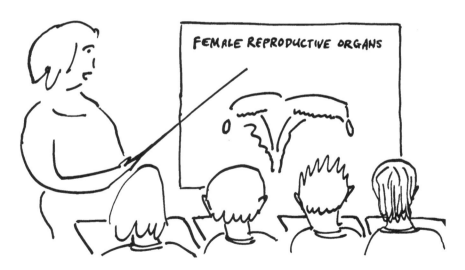

"Excuse me Miss, what does sex feel like?"

My child has an intellectual disability. What should they be learning in sexuality classes?

Children with intellectual disabilities have a right to access honest, accurate and effective information and education about sexuality. It is an unfortunate fact that some children with disabilities are taken advantage of sexually. For their own safety, it is important these children learn about their sexuality. As with other aspects of their learning, they need information repeated in many different ways to enable them to learn.

Parents have a key role in reinforcing the sexuality education program in the school to make the most of this opportunity. If you have a child with an intellectual disability it is important to attend the parents' consultation meetings so that you and your child are able to take full advantage of the program.

A program for primary school children with intellectual disabilities:

1. *Growing up.* The students examine the physical and emotional differences between being a child, teenager and an adult. They also identify the differences between men and women. They name the parts of the body and identify the public and private parts of the body.
2. *Understanding changes at puberty.* The students talk about the changes that take place at puberty.
3. *Public and private.* They identify the public and private places (at home, at school, in the community) and public and private behaviours (toileting, masturbating, showering, getting dressed etc.)
4. *Feelings.* They identify 'yes' feelings and 'no' feelings and the physical signs the body has when they are expressed. They identify the people they can trust and who they could go to for

help. They discuss how inappropriate behaviour can affect others and practise dealing with difficult situations.

5. *Relationships.* They discuss different types of relationships and appropriate and inappropriate touching in those relationships.

Your child may be provided with a workbook and activities they can complete at home. This gives you the opportunity to reinforce the lesson and to incorporate your values. You may be surprised at some of the things we all take for granted, as this story illustrates:

> *Justin came home with his workbook and was asked to find pictures of babies, children, teenagers and adults and talk about how you can tell the difference. We were amazed at how difficult this was for him. He clearly knew what a baby was but otherwise was very unclear about who was a child, teenager or adult. We had told him if he needed help he should ask an adult. We had made the assumption he knew who were adults and who weren't. That was a mistake. We were also surprised that he thought he was the same age as 6 and 7 year olds.*
>
> -Evelyn, mother of Justin, 11 years

Children with intellectual disabilities may be mainstreamed, that is, placed in the same classes as the other children in the school. However their needs are specific and are unlikely to be met if the sexuality education program is not simplified. Schools should provide extra classes in sexuality for them. Where there are only a few students with learning disabilities in the school they could combine classes with other schools in their area.

Be encouraged

Sexuality is a natural and positive part of our lives. It is normal and healthy for people of all ages to have sexual feelings. We all want our children to have loving, caring relationships as adults and to enjoy expressing their sexuality. When young people feel good about themselves and develop good communication skills they are more likely to avoid making mistakes and develop positive, healthy relationships in the future. Sexuality education in schools is one way we can help young people develop the self-esteem and the skills to have honest, open relationships throughout their lives.

Special situations

16

Single parents

I knew I couldn't be both mother and father to my boys. They got on well with their uncle so I asked him to have a man-to-man talk with them. But I checked out where he was coming from so that I knew we had the same ideas about how to treat women and that sort of thing.

Leilani, single mother of three[1]

If you are a single parent you face many more challenges than other parents. Whether you are single because you are separated or divorced, your partner has died, or you have always been a single parent, parenting alone is very demanding. Decisions often need to be made without the opportunity to discuss them with another adult. You may not have the companionship a partner provides. You have less free time for socialisation and relaxation, and usually less money to spend.

Single parents often give their children's needs priority over their own needs.

Elliot felt he had enough on his plate trying to raise his children by himself after his wife died, without contemplating another relationship. He had made a decision not to become emotionally involved with anyone else, mainly because he thought it would be too difficult for the children to accept.

Single parents face situations that married parents don't have to confront. These mainly involve new relationships. Consider these comments from the children of single parents:

> Mum, why do you have such sleazy boyfriends?

Mum, why do you have such sleazy boyfriends?

-Stephanie, 10 years

Dad, the kids at school are teasing me that you are going out with Sarah's Mum.

-Kim, 6 years

I wish you wouldn't go out with that man all the time.

-Francis, 8 years, when her mother dated twice in 10 days

And these comments from single parents:

When Peter is at our house, Jenny is all over him. It's almost like she's flirting with him.

-Win, talking about her new boyfriend and her 5-year-old

I can't come to terms with my ex-husband being gay. I worry that he'll have another man at his house when the kids are there. I try to only let him see them in town. I've tried to get the Court to make it that he can only see them in a public place, but they reckon that's discrimination. I don't care what it is, it just doesn't seem right for the kids.

-Sally, mother of twin boys

We are all very sexual beings. The need for intimacy for a single parent is no less than for parents in a two-parent family. However single parents are aware that a new relationship will have an affect on their child. The key to having your child feel comfortable about a new relationship is to feel comfortable in yourself. If you are happy, relaxed and honest about forming a new friendship your child will pick up those messages from you. If you feel guilty, worried and secretive about a new lover, your child will feel the same way.

> *Jed had had several girlfriends since he left his wife Linda.*
> *He had custody of the children. He always talked about his*
> *relationships with his children and made it clear that if he*
> *met someone he thought he wanted to have a long-term*
> *relationship with he would talk to them before making any*
> *decisions. The children seemed to accept his girlfriends and*
> *did not hesitate to give Jed their opinions of them.*

After a family break-up the single parent will often have less time to spend with their child or children because they no longer have a partner taking their share of the workload. When a new relationship begins, the time a parent can spend with their child is further reduced. Understandably, the child is likely to resent this. This resentment is even stronger when one parent makes derogatory comments about their ex-partner. The child is likely to feel confused and upset.

Following a separation or divorce children often unrealistically dream that there will be reconciliation between the parents. If a parent forms a relationship with someone new the child's dream will be threatened. For this reason the child will resent the new person. This resentment may be expressed by hostility or rejection. The child may express these feelings by constantly criticising the new person, misbehaving, or becoming aggressive toward them.

Conflicting family rules

I find it really hard when Kimberly comes back after being with her Dad because we have different rules to him. When she is here I expect her to help with the jobs and it's like we have to go over it each time she comes back.

-Carolyn, who shares parenting week about with her ex-husband[2]

My ex-wife found that I sometimes had my girlfriend staying overnight on the weekends when I had my kids to stay. She thought that it would somehow harm the children. I reckon it's fine, after all I'm an adult and there's nothing wrong with being in a relationship. But I can't convince my ex-wife, and she is refusing to let the kids stay overnight now. I know that she tells the kids that I'm sleeping around. It's not like that and it's none of her business anyway.

-Finn, father of three

If your child spends time with parents in two separate households they will be faced with different and sometimes conflicting rules and values, different expectations and standards of behaviour.[3] If both parents accept that each household is different and understand that the transition from one to the other won't be easy for the child, the child will adjust more readily.

How can you help your child accept a new relationship?

Children of single parents can find it very difficult to accept that their parent may want to enter a new relationship. If your child is finding it difficult the following suggestions may give you some ideas:

- If they are rude or behave badly towards your new partner take time to talk to them about it. Focus on how they feel rather than their behaviour. You could ask, "Are you feeling angry or worried about something?" If they aren't sure what is upsetting them make a suggestion about what it might be. You could say, "Are you worried that I might love Paul (your new friend) more than you?" or "Are you angry because you want Mummy to come back to live with us?"

- Children need to feel secure, valued and loved. Telling and showing your child that you love them as much now as you did before a family break-up or the death of a spouse will foster those feelings.

- When introducing a new partner to your family it is probably better to do so gradually. This gives everyone time to adjust and get to know each other. It will also be easier for your child if you don't show the affection you have for each other too openly at first.

- Accept that there will be a different set of standards in your ex-partners home, and don't put your ex-partner down when talking to your child. If you have a problem with your ex-partner's behaviour talk to them about it. You child doesn't need to be involved.

- Children need stability. They feel more secure with a routine. Spend a set time every day exclusively with your child. When going out let them know where you are going and when they can expect you to come home again.

- Your new partner may need help to understand your child's behaviour and to cope with your child's rejection. Their constant rejection can be very hurtful and even the best natured person may give up trying to come closer to the child. This could result in the child and the new partner never developing a close, supportive relationship.

- If you are a single parent with a new partner you may also find some of the information in the stepfamilies section of this chapter relevant.

If you are separated or divorced and your ex-partner is responsible for most of your child's care, make sure you don't lose touch with them. Maintaining contact is your responsibility not your child's or the other parent's. It isn't good enough to tell them to phone you when they need to or feel like having a chat. They need to know you care for them enough to call them.

Following a marriage break-up, both parents should continue talking to their child about sexuality issues. Having two very different perspectives about sex, life and relationships is positive. It will help them form their own ideas and develop their own values.

17

Stepfamilies

Stepfamilies are often referred to as 'blended' families. Three or more people come together to form a family which is not their first family. The smallest stepfamily is a stepparent, parent and one child. Relationships in first-time families are complex. However, when two families come together to form a stepfamily the relationships are even more complicated. This chapter addresses the stepfamily issues of showing affection in front of the children, sexual behaviour between stepchildren and differences in attitudes to nudity and privacy.

Displaying affection

When a new stepfamily is formed it can be a confusing time for children. Young children are often not aware of their parent's sexuality in their first-time family. Their parents have over time reduced or stopped kissing, cuddling and being intimate when the children are present. The parents may not have been intimate for some time. In the new stepfamily though, their parent and stepparent are often in the first flush of their new relationship. They touch and kiss each other openly and show more explicit sexual contact than the child can remember from the first-time family.[4]

Have you seen a PDA recently? You probably have. PDA stands for Public Display of Affection, and is a military abbreviation. There are rules in the armed services such as *No PDAs in the Mess*. The reason for this rule is to prevent offence, embarrassment or jealousy amongst the troops. Similarly, your 'troops' may be embarrassed, or upset by their mother or father's amorous behaviour with their new stepparent. Young children may try to physically separate their parent and stepparent when they are hugging, or say things like, "Stop kissing him all the time Mummy".

Stop kissing him all the time Mummy

When Susan (3 years) found her mother June and new stepfather Sam cuddling and kissing in the kitchen, she stood quietly beside them and gently hit Sam on the leg with her fist, but didn't say anything.

This was Susan's way of showing her discomfort with this new relationship. Many young children have similar reactions, and are protective of their parent. It will take time (months or years) before they will be comfortable with the new sexual relationship their parent has entered into.

The child's biological parents may have been separated for some time. During that period they have had one parent to themselves. In the new family the child has to share their parent with their stepparent and possibly other siblings. If their other biological parent has also entered into a new relationship they may feel neglected by both families. When joint custody is involved the child will be spending time with their other stepfamily and stepchildren. It is easy to see how challenging it is for parents and stepparents to help their children adapt to their new families.

How can you help?

In the first months of the new stepfamily limit the amount of touching and kissing you do in front of the children. There are other ways of letting the children know that you love each other. After a few months you can show more physical affection in their presence, as they become familiar with the new stepparent and the new relationship.

Ask the children about their feelings and concerns. Reassure them of your love and continue to give them the love and affection you gave them before. Spending time with each of your children individually is important. They will then have an opportunity to talk about their feelings and any problems they are having.

Sexual behaviour between stepchildren

Sexual behaviour between stepchildren can be an issue when stepfamilies are formed and both new partners have children. Stepfamilies bring together children who are biologically unrelated. However in the new stepfamily all the children are deemed to be related by marriage, whether their parent and stepparent are legally married or not. The children are in fact now brothers and sisters. There is a risk of inappropriate sexual experimentation or activity between stepsiblings.[5] Reasons for this are because they are biologically unrelated, or because they are not familiar with each other, or for a number of emotional and other factors.

It is natural for young children to explore each other's sexual differences in the playful, curious way described in Chapter 7. However a stepparent may feel more anxious if they weren't aware of their child exploring in this way before the new family formed and may feel they are doing something unnatural or harmful. Alternatively they may be in a situation where their new partner accuses their children of aberrant behaviour, after observing sex play between the children. Both parents need to decide whether this is within the range of normal behaviours. Sex play is not usually a problem if all the children are happy and are not being secretive.

There may be a situation where one child may try to do something hurtful or embarrassing to a step-sibling. They may do this in order to punish the new parent or even their own parent, especially if they are feeling left out and confused about the new relationship.

Step-siblings reaching the age of puberty may seek the love and affection from each other that they feel they have lost from their own parent. This can occur easily because they spend a lot of time together and they have a bond because they are going through a similar situation. They may be sexually attracted to each other and this could lead to sexual experimentation. Each child may seek to meet their own needs in what is a very complex situation. One child may be exploited by another. Because the behaviour started with mutual consent they may feel responsible for the situation. They can feel guilty that it is happening but are unable to stop it.

What can you do to help?

At any age a child may try to talk to their own parent about the issues and be rejected for a number of reasons. Some parents don't want to hear that there are conflicts between the children and may feel it is up to the children to sort out their new relationships within the family. The parent may think their child is making up stories, is misinterpreting the situation, or trying to get a sibling into trouble.

If your child is appearing sad, withdrawn, or has had a major change in their behaviour and tries to tell you about a sexual situation, take it seriously. Show them that you are listening and that they are doing the right thing in talking to you. Tell them you won't blame them for whatever is happening and that you will do something about it. Do not hesitate to seek professional advice. In the worst case it may be that your new partner has made sexual advances to your child. Refer to Chapter 18 on *Keeping safe*.

Differences in attitudes to personal matters

As children get older family rules are gradually developed about nudity and privacy. The rules are often unstated and will be different in each family. For example, a family of a mother and two daughters may be very relaxed about privacy.

> *Angela brought up her two daughters Chloe and Rozelle after Angela's husband died when the girls were young. They were very relaxed about privacy. They would think nothing of sharing clothing and walking into the bathroom while each other showered. Angela fell in love with Rubin and he moved in with her, bringing his daughter Corina. Rubin and Corina found the lack of modesty in the new household embarrassing. Corina felt possessive of her clothes and was upset when Chloe and Rozelle helped themselves to her things without asking.*

Angela and her daughters had an established set of family rules about privacy and sharing, and so did Rubin and Corina. When these families came together there was a conflict of rules. Rubin and Corina felt very embarrassed. Corina also felt powerless when the others used her things, as she was in their house and she thought she was expected to fit in with her new sisters. The conflict and embarrassment could have been avoided if they were more aware of each other's family rules and habits.

People living together in a family get to know each other's personal habits, any of which can become annoying. This could be leaving the top off the toothpaste, leaving hair in the basin, or spending a long time in the bathroom. More seriously, people can offend others by being unaware of cultural differences.

For example, for many Maori it is offensive to sit on the table, wash your hands at the kitchen sink, or not to take your shoes off before entering the house. It is a sign of respect to lower your head when talking to someone older, but disrespectful to look them in the eye. This is at odds with Western culture, which values eye contact when talking. Cultural issues such as these will exist in all families with different cultural backgrounds, but are intensified when two families come together to form a stepfamily.

What can you do?

- Try to identify the different cultural practices in the two families that are coming together. This can be difficult because we tend to accept our own cultural customs as 'the way it's done around here'.

- Identify the rules each first-time family had about nudity, privacy, and sharing of possessions before living together. Then establish a new set of rules. You will need to accommodate the most modest child or parent, not reach a compromise. A compromise would not work for the modest member of the family.

18

Keeping safe

When Jonno was six he was sitting on the back seat of the school bus when four high school boys got on and told him to move. He ignored them and looked out the window. They started to rough him up but he managed to slip between them and get to the front. He was upset when he got home, but I was pleased he'd got himself out of danger.

-Travis, father of three

Zara (9 years) had been quiet and moody for a few weeks and I couldn't find out what was wrong. I put it down to the fact her periods had started and she was going through a moody phase. Then one morning she burst into tears saying the boys at school had been teasing her about the size of her breasts and snapping her bra.

-Marguarite, mother of four

You want to keep your child safe in many potentially risky situations. Teaching your toddler the rules of road safety, not to step off the bus or train until it has stopped, and care with electrical appliances are examples. Other risks to their safety are bullying, sexual harassment and sexual abuse. This chapter is about keeping your child safe from sexual harassment and sexual abuse.

Sexual harassment

In the last story the boys at school were verbally and physically harassing Zara. Sexual harassment can happen at any school and at any age. Pushing, shoving, unwanted touching and fondling are common and children learn that harassment happens despite the school policies and rules that may be in place. There are children and adults who will disregard your child's personal boundaries. Sexual harassment can be spoken, written or physical, for example wolf-whistling, making obscene gestures, writing notes, standing too close or unwanted touching. Tell your child they have a right to have their personal space respected, and they can get help to stop harassment. When you are talking about family rules and respecting people's boundaries, suggest ways to respond to people who harass them. Strategies for dealing with sexual harassment and abuse and keeping your child safe are given later in this chapter.

Sexual abuse

Child sexual abuse is a horrific crime. It includes sexual touching, involving children in sexual acts or watching sexual acts. You will have read and heard in the media that social agencies are deeply concerned about child sexual abuse. They encourage people to report incidents or child behaviours that may indicate abuse in an effort to break the cycle of abuse within some families.

Most of us don't want to think about the possibility of our child being sexually abused. When your child is a baby you usually have complete control about whose care they are in. However as they gain more independence they come into contact with a wider range of people and you lose some of that control. Anyone could harm them but they are more likely to be abused by people they know, often in the family or extended family, than by strangers. There is a risk that the people you trust to care for your child may betray that trust. So what can you do to lessen the risk of sexual abuse, without frightening your child?

Recognising unsafe situations

You want your child to be safe. You want to be able to protect them from danger. But the reality is you can't always be there to protect them. Try not to dwell on possible traumatic events when talking to your child about keeping safe. Reassure them that they are unlikely to come into contact with people who would hurt them.[6] Prepare them so that they know what to do if something bad happens. They can learn how to recognise an unsafe situation, learn how to stay in control and what to do to get out of danger.

One way to recognise an unsafe situation is to know the way the body responds when you are scared. Adrenalin is released and the heart beats faster, the blood is redirected to the muscles for action, breathing becomes rapid and you feel alert. When you are in danger the body has one or more 'early warning signs'.[7] For example, your knees feel like jelly, you may have an urge to urinate, palms feel sweaty or you get a feeling of butterflies in the stomach.

Teaching your child to recognise these signs means they can be alert to possible danger. Help them identify these signs by relating them to a scary but safe experience they have had recently. For example, a roller coaster ride or their first time on a water slide. Their physical responses to scary but exciting situations will be the same as scary but unsafe traumatic events.

What can they do when they sense danger?

When their early warning signs alert them something is wrong they need to take action. Tell them if someone is doing something that makes them feel scared they could move away, tell the person to stop or get someone to help them. Give them ideas such as yelling or doing something gross to distract the person. For example, spitting or pretending to vomit will give them time to get away. Tell them that these are only suggestions and they have your permission to do anything they can at the time.

Ella, 10 years, liked her cousin Mike coming to babysit. He let her stay up late and watch TV programs her mother wouldn't let her watch. But one night he moved very close to her and put his arm along the back of the couch behind her. He said he could see she was growing up. He put his hand on her breast 'to see how big she was getting'. She felt so scared that her throat went tight and dry. When she tried to tell him to stop no sound came out. She pushed him away, ran into her mother's room and locked the door. Feeling safe she then used the phone beside the bed to ring the next door neighbour.

Ella had acted on her 'early warning sign'. In this case her throat felt tight and dry. Her mother had talked to her about how her body felt when she was scared. Ella had said her throat had felt tight and dry when she had watched a scary movie. When Mike had touched her she recognised she was in danger and needed to do something. Ella had acted early and was safe.

Child sexual abuse is abhorrent. Unfortunately it is easy to pass on your horror and fear of it when talking to your child. Passing your feelings of fear and anxiety to them is not helpful. We can't frighten children into feeling safe. The best way to protect your child from sexual abuse is to build their inner strength and self-confidence so that in the event of potential abuse they will not feel powerless and will know what to do.

What can you do to help your child keep safe?

There are many skills your child can learn from you to help them stay safe. Giving them these skills before they reach puberty is your responsibility. Even if your child's school has a good program about keeping safe, don't rely on the school to do it for you. Parents are the first and most important teachers, and your child needs to learn about keeping safe from you. Try some of these suggestions:

- Teach them that the private parts of their body are special and that no one can look at or touch those parts without their permission.
- Help them identify at least one early warning sign. These are the first ways our bodies tell us that we are not feeling safe. They are physical sensations. Examples of early warning signs are: their legs feel like jelly, their throat feels tight and dry, their heart starts pounding or their stomach feels funny.
- Use fairytales to talk about early warning signs. For example you may be telling the story about 'The three little pigs.' You could ask "How does the little pig feel when the wolf is outside huffing and puffing and trying to blow the little pig's house down? What are his early warning signs?"
- Help them identify people they know they can trust. They could be in the family, at their preschool or school, or in the community. These are the people to talk to if they are worried or in trouble.
- As your child goes through puberty they need to have other trusted adults they can talk to. At this age it becomes more difficult for a father to fill this role with his son. Make sure boys know other men care for them throughout their lives - an uncle, or coach, a male teacher, or a family friend.
- Find out what sexuality education your child's school is providing and see what you can do to support it. Young people need to have the confidence to enjoy early sexual feelings without going on to have sexual intercourse. Sexuality education at puberty will help them do this.
- You could take action to support sexuality education at your school. You may also be in a position to develop policies that address sexuality issues.
- Don't withdraw the natural affection and intimacy that you share with your child for fear of unfairly being accused of sexual abuse.

- Don't expect your child to kiss, hug or sit on someone's lap if they don't want to.

What is sexual abuse?

Using a child for sexual pleasure is sexual abuse. Sexual abuse includes performing sexual acts with a child; touching a child sexually over or under clothing; a child being coerced or tricked into touching the sexual parts of another person; a child being forced to watch adults touching the sexual parts of their bodies; a child being exposed to pornography or being photographed for pornographic materials. In New Zealand and in most Western countries it is illegal for any adult to have sex or commit sexual acts with a child under 16 years old.

A child who is sexually abused often knows the abuser, who may be a relative or a friend of the family. The abuse is most likely to develop gradually over time, and the incidents of abuse may occur on more than one occasion.

Children who are forced to watch others have sex are being abused. It is also unhealthy for children to be constantly exposed to abusive adult sexual behaviour. Some children see or hear violent sexual activity in their own family. It may be part of their everyday lives. These children are not sure what is going on. They may feel frightened or excited by it or worry that the adults are hurting each other. They become confused about what is normal and what is not. They become confused about what is appropriate and what is not.

Feeling guilty

When people are sexually abused they may feel guilty, confused, scared and powerless. They may have been enjoying the initial contact with the abuser and believe they encouraged the abuse, and feel it was their own fault. The abuser has more authority than the child and often tells them not to tell anyone about what they are doing. It is their secret and if they tell they will get into trouble or something bad will happen to someone they love. The child may like the abuser and want to protect them, even though they don't like the abuse.

If someone mistreats your child you want to know. Reassure them that there is nothing too terrible they can't tell you.

What should you do if you suspect abuse?

In the event of your child telling you something you suspect may be abuse, don't panic or overreact. You can:

- tell your child you are pleased they told you
- tell them that it is not their fault
- reassure them you love them
- tell them you will get help to sort it out

If you suspect your child has been sexually abused you need to get professional help from a doctor or health worker trained in dealing with child sexual abuse. Don't repeatedly ask them what happened or ask for too much detail. If they are asked lots of questions children can get confused about what actually happened. Leave the interviewing to the professionals.

Fathers and intimacy

Larry cared for his daughter Kate during the day, fitting his work on their farm around the time she was at kindergarten. Sometimes Kate asked her friend Vicky to come and play at her house. Larry became aware that Vicky's mother was hesitating to agree to this. He sensed her anxiety about having them alone with him on the farm. He became fearful that if Vicky's mother accused him of wrongdoing he would have no witnesses to support him. He made a decision not to have other children to play at home with Kate unless another adult was present.

Men like Larry who care for children alone may feel they need to be more cautious when their children's friends come home to play. Larry decided to make sure other adults were present when Kate had her friends home to play. He could also have talked to Vicky's mother about her fears. Larry is a great role model for Kate and her friends in his caring for the children and it would be beneficial for all of them if he continued. Talking about it to other men who are in a similar situation would also be helpful.

People have become increasingly aware of child abuse and many agencies are working together to identify and reduce the problem. Fathers need to be aware that there have been cases in which a father's behaviour has been misinterpreted and false allegations of sexual abuse made. Unfortunately this possibility has caused some fathers to withdraw the intimacy they have previously enjoyed with their children. This in turn has a negative effect on the relationship between the father and his child. It also reinforces the male stereotype that men are not as competent as women in the nurturing and caring role for children. It is very important that you as a father continue to show affection to your child and take a positive role in the caring of your child.

Sexual behaviour between children as young as 12 years old

Sexual intercourse or sexual activity such as oral sex before the age of twelve is sexual abuse. It is abuse when the abuser is older than the child but it is also abuse when it occurs between children of the same age. For some children the abusive behaviour they are exposed to at home is reflected in their own activity.

A study conducted in the Hawke's Bay region of New Zealand found that one in eight 14-year-olds reported having first sex at age twelve or younger.[8] Twenty percent of these sexually active young people were reporting they had had more than five sexual partners by age 14. Having multiple sexual partners puts these young people at high risk of sexually transmissible infections and unintended pregnancy. Most of the boys in the study did not know if their girlfriends were using contraception. These young people were involved in activity that could have had life-changing consequences. Twelve-year-olds should not be having sex. They aren't mature enough - emotionally, physically or socially.

People who work with adolescents hear from them that young people who start having sex before they are sixteen say they should have waited longer. They say their early sexual experiences have often been negative and they were under pressure at the time. It left them confused and feeling bad about themselves. When a person's self-esteem is shaken they are less able to make healthy decisions, often leading to further problems.

What can parents do?

Most of the sexually active young people in the study didn't think their parents knew they were having sex. Many of them said they would have liked to have been able to ask their mothers for their advice. To avoid your child being in this situation you need to talk about sexual matters well before they are twelve and let them know you are always there for them. Stay in touch with what they are doing and the people they are spending time with. Children need a clear message that twelve years old is far too young for intimate sexual behaviour.

Endnotes

19

Your success

Imagine the day your child becomes a teenager – their thirteenth birthday. We want to congratulate you in advance. You are giving your child a great start to their life. You see sexual development as a positive, natural part of their growing up, and you have been teaching them informally about their sexuality since they were born. There won't been a need for the 'Big Talk' at puberty because you will have dealt with sexuality issues naturally and with confidence during their childhood. You will have laid a sound foundation for what may be the turmoil of adolescence. The values, knowledge and skills your child is developing will give them confidence as they navigate those sometimes stormy waters.

Parenting is hard work. Children can be frustrating, annoying and exasperating. They require endless patience, money and energy. Raising children can be the most demanding yet most important job of a lifetime. The rewards are in watching them grow and develop and in your relationship with them as they move toward becoming independent adults. All parents can think of times they have overreacted, missed opportunities, said the 'wrong' thing or behaved in a way that in retrospect wasn't the behaviour of a model parent. However children are extremely resilient and very forgiving. Treat them with love and respect and you will be rewarded.

We are sure you have enjoyed the stories we have shared with you. You have your own stories. If you share them with other parents they will appreciate your openness. You can help them gain the same confidence you have developed through your own parenting.

We wish you well for the future as you guide your child through adolescence. The work you have done means they feel good about themselves and can express feelings of affection, love and intimacy as they mature. The healthy sexuality values and attitudes you are helping them develop will prepare them for committed loving relationships as adults.

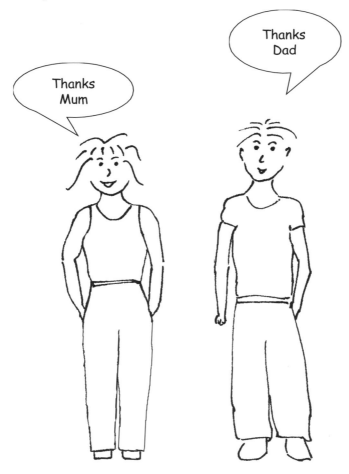

Notes and references

Getting started

1. Quoted in Lusk, B. (1999). *Making a difference - a guide for health co-ordinators and teachers.* Wellington: NZFPA.
2. Ibid.
3. Legge, K. (1997, December 14). Child's play beyond the cabbage patch. *Sunday Star-Times.* p. 11.
4. Zilbergeld, B. (1993). *The new male sexuality.* New York: Bantam Books
5. Rothbaum, F., Grauer, A., & Rubin, D. (1997). Becoming sexual: Differences between child and adult sexuality. *Young Children, 52(6)*, 22-28.
6. Dear Barbie Mag. (2001, March). *Barbie, 54*, p. 31.
7. Based on New Zealand Family Planning Association sexuality workshops for parents.

Children's sexual development

1. Levitt, S. (Ed.). (1994). *Paediatric developmental therapy.* Oxford: Blackwell Scientific.
2. Marieb, E. (1997). *Human anatomy and physiology.* Redwood City, CA: Benjamin Cummings.
3. Illingworth, R., & Dubowitz, V. (1991). *The normal child.* Edinburgh: Churchill Livingston.
4. Levitt, S. (Ed.). (1994). *Paediatric developmental therapy.* Oxford: Blackwell Scientific.

5. Goldman, R. & J. (1982). *Children's sexual thinking.* London: Routledge & Kegan Paul.
6. Early Childhood Sexuality Education Taskforce. (1995). *Right from the start: Guidelines for sexuality issues.* New York: SIECUS.
7. Rothbaum, F., Grauer, A., & Rubin, D. (1997). Becoming sexual: Differences between child and adult sexuality. *Young Children, 52(6)*, 22-28
8. Goldman, R. & J. (1982). *Children's sexual thinking.* London: Routledge & Kegan Paul.
9. New Zealand Ministry of Education. (1993). *Te whariki.* Wellington: Learning Media.
10. Wilson, P. (1991). *When sex is the subject.* Santa Cruz, CA: Network Publications.
11. Lough, G. (2000). *Parents – talking with your kids about sex.* Wellington: NZFPA.
12. Hoffman, L., Paris, S., & Hall, E. (1993). *Developmental psychology today.* NY: McGraw-Hill
13. Rudolf, M., & Levene, M. (1998). *Paediatrics & child health.* Oxford: Blackwell Science.
14. University of Auckland. (1984). *Misconceptions.* Video. Auckland: University of Auckland.
15. Ibid.
16. Rudolf, M., & Levene, M. (1998). *Paediatrics & child health.* Oxford: Blackwell Science.
17. Ibid.

18. Wilson, P. (1991). *When sex is the subject.* Santa Cruz, CA: Network Publications.
19. St. George et al (1994). Dunedin Multidisciplinary Health and Development Study. In New Zealand Ministry of Health: *Our children's health.*
20. Biddulph, S. (1998). *Raising boys.* Berkeley, CA: Celestial Arts.
21. Gray, J., & Jilich, J. (1990). *Janet's got her period.* Australia.
22. More girls reaching puberty by age eight. (2000, June 19). *The Dominion,* p. 5.
23. Cleland, A., & Mackay, L.. (1994). *A study of the effectiveness of sexuality education programs.* Auckland: University of Auckland.
24. New Zealand Department of Internal Affairs. (2000). *Online safety.* Wellington: DIA.

Ask me anything

1. Rothbaum, F., Grauer, A., & Rubin, D. (1997). Becoming sexual: Differences between child and adult sexuality. *Young Children, 52(6),* 22-28.
2. Sex Information and Education Council of the US. (2000, November 13). www.siecus.com
3. New Zealand Mental Health Foundation. (1996). *Good communication.* Wellington: Ministry of Health.
4. Family planning Association of New Zealand. (1996). *Grab that moment.* Wellington: FPANZ.
5. We have applied a step-by-step process adapted from SIECUS. You can find further examples on www.siecus.com
6. Norfor, J. *Communication: Relating assertively with others.* Sydney: Western Sydney Area Health Promotion Centre.
7. Hoffman, L., Paris, S., & Hall, E. (1993). *Developmental psychology today.* NY: McGraw-Hill.
8. Newman, M. (1992). *Stepfamily realities.* Sydney: Doubleday.
9. Early Childhood Sexuality Education Taskforce. (1995). *Right from the start: Guidelines for sexuality issues.* New York: SIECUS.

At School

1. The information in *At School* is based on 12 years personal experience of supporting the implementation of sexuality education in schools in New Zealand. This included training teachers, teaching the students when teachers have felt lacking in the skills to teach the material themselves, assisting with the planning of programs, providing resources, talking to parents at parent consultation meetings and at parent workshops, consulting young people about what they want to know and assessing their present knowledge.
2. Lusk, B. (1999). Making a difference - a guide for health co-ordinators and teachers. Wellington: NZFPA.
3. Rothbaum, F., Grauer, A., & Rubin, D. (1997). Becoming sexual: Differences between child and adult sexuality. *Young Children, 52(6),* 22-28.
4. Lusk, B. (1999). Making a difference - a guide for health co-ordinators and teachers. Wellington: NZFPA.
5. Parents want school sex education. (2000, December 30). *The Dominion,* p. 3.
6. Cleland, A., & Mackay, L.. (1994). *A study of the effectiveness of sexuality education programmes.* Auckland: University of Auckland

7. Kirby, D. (1994). *School-based programs to reduce sexual risk behaviours: A review of effectiveness.* ETR Associates.
8. National Guidelines Task Force. (1994). *Guidelines for comprehensive sexuality education.* New York: Sex Information and Education Council of the US.
9. New Zealand Ministry of Education. (1999). *The New Zealand Health and Physical Education Curriculum.* Wellington: Learning Media.
10. Brown, S.(1993). *Streetwise to sexwise.* Hackensack, NJ: Center for Family Life Education. Activity adapted from sexual decision making strategy.

Special situations

1. Lough, G. (2000). *Parents – talking with your kids about sex.* Wellington: NZFPA.
2. Ibid.
3. Wattleton, F. & Keiffer, E. (1986). *How to talk with your child about sexuality.* New York: Doubleday.
4. Newman, M. (1992). *Stepfamily realities.* Sydney: Doubleday.
5. Ibid.
6. Jacobs, D., & Jacobs, R. (1999). *Zip your lips.* Boston: Element Books.
7. Flandreau West, P.(1989). *The Basic Essentials.* Burnside, SA: Essence Training.
8. Fenwicke, R. (2000). The sexual activity of 654 fourth form Hawke's Bay students. *New Zealand Medical Journal 113*, 460-463.

Further reading

For parents

Bernstein, A. (1994). *Flight of the stork.* Chicago: Perspective.

Biddulph, S. (1998). *Raising boys.* Berkeley, CA: Celestial Arts.

Calderone, M.S., & Ramey, J.W. (1982). *Talking with your child about sex.* NewYork: Random House.

Constantine, L. & Martinson, F. (1981). *Children and sex: New findings, new perspectives.* Boston: Little, Brown.

Goldman, R. & J. (1982). *Children's sexual thinking.* London: Routledge & Kegan Paul.

Gordon, S., & J. Gordon. (1989). *Raising a child conservatively in a sexually permissive world.* New York: Simon & Schuster.

Jacobs, D, & Jacobs, R. (1999). *Zip your lips.* Boston: Element Books.

Kotzman, A. (1989). *Listen to me listen to you.* Melbourne: Penguin.

Leight, L. (1990). *Raising sexually healthy children.* New York: Avon.

Linke, P. (1997). *Pants aren't rude.* Canberra: Goanna Print.

Lively, V. (1991). *Sexual development of young children.* Albany, NY: Delmar.

Lough, G. (2000). *Parents – talking with your kids about sex.* Wellington: NZFPA.

Newman, M. (1992). *Stepfamily realities.* Sydney: Doubleday.

Rothbaum, F., Grauer, A., & Rubin, D. (1997). Becoming sexual: Differences between child and adult sexuality. *Young Children, 52(6),* 22-28.

Shakespeare, T., Gillespie, K., Sells & Davies, D. (1996). *The sexual politics of disability.* London & New York: Cassell

Wattleton, F. & Keiffer, E. (1986). *How to talk with your child about sexuality.* New York: Doubleday.

Wilson, P. (1991). *When sex is the subject.* Santa Cruz, CA: ETR Associates.

For children

Brooks, R. (1983). *So that's how I was born!* New York: Simon & Schuster.

Cooke, K. (1994). *Real Gorgeous.* NSW: Allen and Unwin.

Freeman, L. (1995). *It's my body.* NSW: Pademelon Press.

Harris, R. (1994). *It's perfectly normal: Changing bodies, growing up, sex and sexual health.* Cambridge, MA: Candlewick.

Mayle, P. (1990). *Where did I come from?* 2d ed. New York: Carol.

Patterson, C., & Quilter, L. (1990). *It's OK to be you!* Wellington: Random House Publishing.

Schoen, M. (1990). *Belly buttons are navels.* Amherst, NY: Prometheus.

Stinson, C. (1997). *The bare naked book.* Toronto: Annick.

Index

Order Form

Please send me:
_____ copies *From Birth to Puberty*   NZ$21.95   AUS$21.95

Total including free postage and packing (Australasia) _____

For prices for the rest of the world visit www.frombirthtopuberty.com

Please make cheques payable to Suntime and cross 'Not Transferable'

Name   _____

Address   _____

        _____

        _____

email: (for confirmation of order)_____

Organizations may pay on invoice when goods are supplied

Post to:
Suntime,
PO Box 5158 Greenmeadows
Napier, New Zealand

Secure credit card payment is available, email suntime@paradise.net.nz
for details. For security reasons, do not email your credit card number.

Thank you for your order

http://www.frombirthtopuberty.com/

From Birth to Puberty